You Are
HOW
YOU
MOVE

GED SUMNER

You Are HOW YOU MOVE

Experiential Chi Kung

SINGING DRAGON
London and Philadelphia

Exercises in this book can be followed online at: www.naturalmovement.info

First published in 2009
by Singing Dragon
An imprint of Jessica Kingsley Publishers
116 Pentonville Road
London N1 9JB, UK
and
400 Market Street, Suite 400
Philadelphia, PA 19106, USA

www.singing-dragon.com

Copyright © Ged Sumner 2009

Library of Congress Cataloging in Publication Data
A CIP catalog record for this book is available from the Library of Congress

British Library Cataloguing in Publication Data
A CIP catalogue record for this book is available from the British Library

ISBN 978 1 84819 014 6

Printed and bound in the United States by
Thomson-Shore, 7300 Joy Road, Dexter, MI 48130

CONTENTS

ACKNOWLEDGMENTS

Many thanks to the following people for giving up their time to be photographed: Ute Stenger, Jenny and Lyla Keogh, and Kim Michelle. Thank you to Chris O'Kane for taking many of the pictures, and Belinda Ackermann for taking some pictures. Deepest thanks go to Manuela Viana for her valuable and intelligent contributions to editing the book.

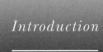

WHAT IS EXERCISE?

Ask people the question "What is exercise?" and you might find yourself getting remarkably consistent feedback. "Exercise" seems to generate images of humans engaged in strong physical activity such as sports, running, aerobics and workouts on machines at the gym. The picture of faces strained by physical exertion comes to mind, with varying degrees of enthusiasm. Few people regard warming up and stretching as an important factor, and some suggest that "exercise" is about creating stamina. It's an interesting question to ask, and on the whole most people seem to think that "exercise" is synonymous with "going to the gym".

Then, there's the question of fitness. It seems that the ideal image or goal of exercising is to try to gain some approximation, if only a mediocre one, of the professional athlete at the peak of their performance. Whilst we may all have somewhat disappointed, but perhaps more realistic, understandings of our own limitations, at the back of our minds still lies the image of the perfect human form in peak fitness and performance. Surely there's nothing wrong in aiming for perfection? We all love to watch our supernatural heroes battle through every physical, psychological and emotional challenge to be the best, the ultimate Olympian champion. We all hold this gargantuan physical exertion in the highest regard, whether we are sport oriented or not.

It is inspiring to watch the skill, dedication, determination, talent and well-oiled synchronization of the human form all come together in an athlete to achieve an Olympic medal. In this arena the seemingly impossible suddenly becomes possible. It is here that the image of the "perfect body" enters our psyches and we set about unconsciously trying to achieve that dream body.

Hard-driven exercise might suit some people, but chasing an ideal image, fantasizing about producing a particular body look, losing weight and having a physical performance level that is only possible through tremendous effort is generally unattainable for most people, owing to the lack of time, motivation and dedication necessary. It immediately feels easier to give up before one even begins, for that "perfect body" image is set so high. Rather than become despondent, let's challenge the status quo and question our ideas of exercise and perhaps discover an easier, effective, attainable and enjoyable form of exercise.

It's no wonder that, when most of us consider the idea of exercise, it tends to make us feel immediately stressed. The idea of corporate-looking gyms, drilling exercise regimes, peer pressure and body image start to spoil the mind. That's enough to stop many people from even starting and who can blame them? It does feel exhausting and over-demanding. The old maxim commands "No pain, no gain", indicating that exercise in Western society is associated with enormous effort, and physical pain and strain.

The problem is that most exercise is focused on "looking good" and, in order to achieve this, having to pursue a monotonous exercise regime that doesn't fill you with inspiration, but gets results. The concept of simply feeling good, connected and healthy is of secondary concern. Unfortunately, many people don't realize there's an alternative; so, feeling unfulfilled at the gym, they either stop and start – never really getting into it – or persist and renew their membership, hoping that that will be enough of a motivation, but then don't turn up for weeks and feel guilty; or, exasperated and simply bored, stop exercising altogether, which will probably result in a total lack of movement and therefore lead to poor health.

Statistics say that most people don't exercise consistently beyond the age of thirty, beyond forty less than thirty per cent of the population are exercising at all, and increasingly people are becoming more sedentary each year. It's not hard to miss. Children are driven to school, adults travel in cars and trains, people watch television, spend more time browsing on the internet and play more computer games than ever before, and all this does is help their blood collect in their legs. We don't walk any more and most people are eating nutritionally poor diets or are overweight. In an age where you can eat excellent nutritional food, many people are still eating too much fat, sugar and salt, increasing their bulk and decreasing their metabolism. Western society is so wealthy there's actually an excess of food for the first time in the history of man, as well as the greatest variety of foodstuffs ever imaginable. The choice is so great it's overwhelming. Despite the greatest wealth of intelligent literature and guidance on nutrition that has ever been available, the majority of people are poisoning themselves thanks to lack of food education and poor diet, while the rest of the world is malnourished from the lack of food.

EXERCISE TRAUMA

In modern-day society there's an overwhelming tendency for everything to be stressful. Our basic activities in a day seem to be cloaked with an arrangement of stressful experiences; simple tasks are entangled with frustrating or challenging events and, unfortunately, our body is implicated in all this stress. It reveals this through its basic functioning – from going to the loo, eating and drinking, to discomfort when exercising. Millions of people suffer from constipation, irritable bowels, chronic fatigue, poor nutrition, dehydration, obesity or poor body tone. Commonly, many of these symptoms go hand in hand. It's the sign of the times and a sign that a society is unhealthy. People are simply not coping with modern life and their bodies are suffering. Is it any wonder that depression is the biggest pathology of our time and Prozac one of the most prescribed drugs?

Given that modern life is filled with so many challenges, why is it that, to wind down from an adrenalized day, people force their bodies past their exhaustion and pain thresholds simply to complete the next twelve sets of a workout? In reality, you are driving your body into exhaustion, and that's considered relaxation? Exercise regimes range from obsessively strengthening muscles and firming up with rigorous movement and weight training, to increasing cardiovascular output through running or high exertion. Does the body really enjoy being driven or does it feel like a strain? This method of exercise seems to be all about pushing the body, performing to a greater level and, at its core, it's about competitiveness. Competing with yourself or others, pushing your limits, trying to achieve greater speed, endurance or strength and smashing personal bests. Where did all this come from? Surely this only adds pressure to exercise, orienting towards performance and achievement rather than the good things, such as balance, increased mobility, litheness, feeling uplifted, relaxed and centred.

For example, what is this obsession with running? How good, in fact, is running for the body? There seems to be no purpose to running; runners are not skilfully stalking or hunting prey and neither are they running from danger. On a physical level they are expressing the instinctual response of the primal "flight mode" of survival. The body experiences it as such, but for no real reason, as there is no real threat. Is it such a good idea to place the body into such a state of alert? Actually this heightened state is exhausting for the body. You don't see animals randomly going for a jog around the block. The high that comes from running is triggered by adrenalin, the very stuff that puts you into alert mode. It's definitely not healthy; it's not something that's meant to be turned on all the time. It's there as an immediate response to danger and is therefore meant to be short-term. Once you've dealt with the threat, the natural response would be to move back towards a state of ease. However, that's not what happens in modern life. If you consider that this adrenalized state is already reminiscent of the state of stress you are in, from having to respond to the demands at work, home and general life, going for that thirty-minute steep incline at your personal best is actually just a further addition to the stress. Problems occur when this build-up of stress turns into long-term stress and it has serious consequences for health; that's when illness or exhaustion sets in.

Whilst we criticize the concept of exercise, there is also the age-old condition of people exercising incorrectly by not starting slowly and properly warming up first. It seems people detach from their bodies, do not enter into a state of body awareness, and therefore ignore any in-built signals that inform them of when they might feel strain or be overwhelmed. We are not educated to develop this innate ability. There's nothing more painful or bewildering than watching a middle-aged person running around a park, almost dying from the exertion of it, and running without skill, proper posture or style. You can see their joints getting damaged, not to mention the terrible strain on their heart and lungs. Stop, for God's sake – don't do this to your body! By all means get fit and healthy, but not in this way! This is the way to kill yourself or land up in hospital. The point is, that if you don't find appropriate ways to exercise that make you feel good, you will naturally stop and revert to doing nothing, leading again to a sedentary and unhealthy lifestyle. Why not exercise by learning how to walk – never mind running! Believe it or not, when you begin to walk intelligently, it teaches you how to stand properly – and we could all make better use of that. That's what this book is about, it's about addressing these simple issues of standing, sitting, walking and breathing and exploring them in greater detail so that you can re-invent and reframe what exercise means to you.

WHERE TO START

The good news – an alternative way to exercise

Get wise. Be gentle with yourself. Love your body. Start with soft, easy exercise where you don't have to strain. Simple movements. Exercise can be just as effective and powerful whilst being natural, easy and enjoyable. Yes, easy, not difficult. Easy, meaning no strain or huge effort. Can you believe that there is such a thing as easy exercise that produces results? It's true. Here's a secret.

Focus on loosening your joints. That's it. Just stay with that for a few months. Develop an understanding of all your joints in your body. Spend time investigating how they connect your body up, how many there are, and how much they need to communicate with structures around them. Develop an internal rapport with them. Work out what movements support them, as opposed to putting them under strain. Make your joints your own personal study for a few months. Once you've worked out how they function, what movements work best for them, see if you can synchronize your breath with your movements. Now try the same posture but this time take the hands as far apart as possible so that one hand is below the pelvis with the palm looking down and the other is above the head with the palm looking up. Notice how this affects your general state of being, and how your body can move towards a deep state of rest by simple focused attention. You might find it surprising how much information there is to absorb, and it will be a fascinating and deeply personal discovery.

So the good news is that you don't need to run around the park in a ragged way, straining your body. You can do simple, natural movements/forms that bring suppleness, energy and alacrity to you. Suddenly exercise is open to everyone of any age, not just young or desperate people down at the gym.

So why exercise?

We exercise to optimize our health. Exercising in a natural way, that reduces high impact on the body, will keep you supple and increase your chances of a long, healthy life. This is not just about living long, but living life with health and with all our faculties in place. Contracted bodies don't give rise to clarity and happiness. Erect posture and suppleness means you will have a brain like that. You won't curl up and implode in old age as so many people do. Most people don't ever exercise effectively in their lives, nor eat healthily. So imagine if you did both of these things consistently throughout your life, how would you be at eighty or ninety? It's not such a difficult secret to discover about long life and health. Challenge your perception of what aging means to you. Is it necessary to wither and fade into the background of society? How many people do you know aged seventy who look bright and robust? It's perfectly possible. It's not simply about good luck or strong constitutions. We all have to manage our health and condition to some degree. We either do it well through a good diet and exercise, thereby optimizing our vitality, or we ignore ourselves, and diminish our health with excess drinking, smoking, eating, and any number of over-indulgent practices.

The truth is that the potential for super-health is available to everyone. Here's the formula:

- optimize your diet

- do consistent intelligent exercise

- create the right pacing in your life that brings about internal balance

- avoid stress, poor diet and being sedentary.

Here's the challenge:

Dare to be really healthy! That's it. Ask yourself, are you scared of this state? What is the resistance to being healthy? Why is this the last thing on the agenda? Why do most people insist on poisoning themselves and being in a lethargic state?

Be courageous and become healthy. It means you will almost certainly feel the following things:

- happy
- relaxed
- confident
- creative
- clear
- light.

All that's needed to bring about a sense of well-being is an intelligent diet and intelligent exercise. Here's the exercise bit.

NATURAL MOVEMENT – EXPERIENCING CHI KUNG

What are people trying to achieve from a workout? It seems all that intensity condenses the body even further, adding to the overall compression of our lives. Is it really worth having tight muscles? That euphoric feeling can just as easily be achieved through natural movement. Natural movement is what the body likes to do instinctively. You will feel light and spacious from relieving places of tension, mobilizing joints, and connecting with the body through its connective tissue framework. Physiologically, all of this increases fluid exchange, which is critical to the body's well-being. Energy-wise, it increases the flow and amount of energy available. It balances emotions and creates clarity of mind. Not bad – and all of this can happen gently and quickly. After all, what do tight muscles do to our joints? Why not focus on our joints for a change and engage in movements that warm them up? After all, joints are critical places that affect many systems of the body.

Chi Kung is a science of exercise and internal awareness that produces super-health. Its movements are natural and do not force the body to exceed its capabilities. The movements and internal exercises create a balanced posture and alignment in the body. The body becomes strong through developing an internal strength rather than through muscle power or aerobic activity: quite the opposite of the way we approach exercising the body in the West.

Chi Kung is an ancient Chinese form of movement exercise that promotes the flow of Chi (vital energy) through the body. It translates as "energy work" in English and comprises exercises for stretching and mobilizing the body and joints, breathing techniques, slow movement exercises, static postures, special walking methods and meditation. Chi is the body's vital energy, which the practice of Chi Kung builds up to establish a physiological and psychological harmony.

Chi Kung's origins are a mixture of several traditions. One of the most influential is Traditional Chinese Medicine – Chinese doctors used to commonly prescribe Chi Kung exercises as part of their health advice. A branch of Chi Kung has developed from this, called Medical Chi Kung, that focuses on using prescribed exercises for a variety of health conditions.

Chi Kung is also associated with Taoist and Buddhist philosophies and practices, particularly Taoist. This applies to the internal soft forms of Chi Kung that have their focus on spiritual growth and development through meditation practices. The Taoist element lends a strand of shamanistic theories and practices.

Chi Kung can also be focused on building external Chi. These forms are to be found in association with martial arts.

Chi Kung generally does not have complex "forms". Chi Kung movements are simple. Each action aims to move Chi in a specific way. The forms often take their inspiration from the movement of animals and nature, and can look very elegant. Sometimes the movements follow energy channels in the body, and sometimes they orient around internal organs or parts of the body. The aim in all the movements is to increase the flow of Chi through the mind and body.

The Chi Kung approach in this book is Elemental Chi Kung, which is a progressive approach to Chi Kung that incorporates classic styles and philosophies with modern body–mind and energy concepts. The approach explores body and Chi awareness as a way to deepen into our internal Chi flow through movement, stillness, meditation, and breath. A creative space is sought to allow our essential nature to express itself and bring about transformation at an innermost reality.

Chapter 1

FINDING YOUR SPINE

The largest structure in your body is your spine. It has a huge presence. It's composed of hundreds of individual structures all brought together into a single unit of function of bones, joints, nerves and muscles, that creates a central axis for our body's movements. When it functions healthily, movements will be fluid and supple not just through the spine, but throughout the whole body. Simply becoming aware of your spine can start a process of bringing your spine into a higher state of health. We generally are unaware of our spine until something goes wrong with it. We tend to move around oblivious of its presence, either because we are so used to it that we don't distinguish it from the rest of our body or we are just not that body-aware. The thing about your spine is that when you are sensitive to its movements it becomes a wonderful agile, intelligent phenomenon that truly connects your brain to your body and organizes your body movements with a marvellous orchestration. You can quickly feel the truth of this when you spend time with your spine. Try this movement:

It's a simple movement that should allow your spine to warm up by twisting along its length. Relax your shoulders and let your arms become heavy. Make sure your knees are flexed and knee-caps looking forward. Keeping your spine vertical, let it twist along its length. You will find a natural rhythm in the movement

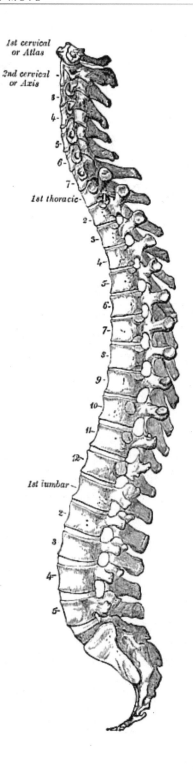

Spine

that is enjoyable and freeing up. Mechanically, it warms up the joints and muscles, but it does much more than that. It brings you into a fuller relationship with your spine and, as you practise this exercise, you'll begin to feel how the spine connects up along its whole length. As each vertebra talks to the next, so the whole spine starts to converse, and it can truly come to know itself as a whole unit of function, and not just a set of individual units orienting around their immediate space. The spine is like a collective, a bit like an organization or family or society. When there's communication, there's awareness of the whole.

Try a variation of this movement by allowing your hands to tap gently on your kidneys at the back of your waist as they reach the end of the swing. This will deepen the twist. When you do

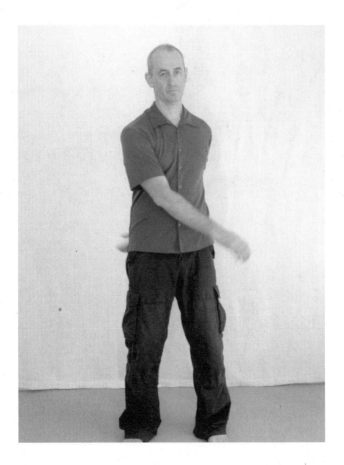

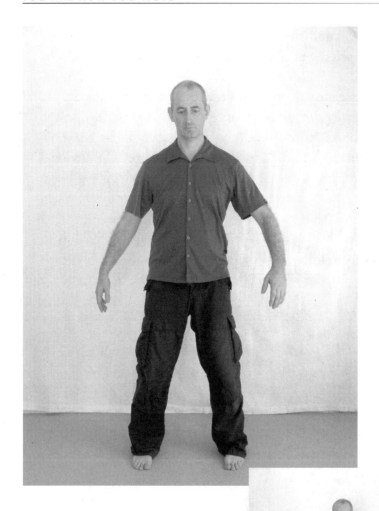

this exercise you will not only feel your spine waking up and becoming more present, but you will quickly feel any place of strain or discomfort, along with places that feel strong and easy. These places can vary from person to person; however, the most common places of strain are the lower back and neck, as well as between the shoulder blades, which can often feel tight and immobile. Draw a picture of your spine and mark on it the places that feel great, as well as the places that are painful or tight. Don't lose touch with the places that feel good. We tend to ignore those and focus on the pain. Doing this will reduce your connection to the spine as a whole, and along with it goes the power and energy of the whole. It's worth thinking about that for a while, as there are profound implications. Losing touch with the places that feel good is losing touch with a lot of your health, vitality and oneness. A downward spiral happens when you get lost in pain and discomfort. Try it and see. Another way to connect with your spine is to bring the hands to the top and bottom of the spine so that the palms look at each other.

Imagine that you are holding the spine in two places. Keep your body as still as you can and make sure your feet are parallel and your knees are not locked. The hold will quickly bring you into a sense of your spine. Stay still for a few minutes and notice what kinds of movements are taking place in your body. Then try moving your hands to different places along the spine and see how that changes things. If you practise this enough times you will become stronger in your spine and have more energy. Here's another exercise that will bring lots of energy to your spine.

Free your spine and the rest of the body will follow. This should be a maxim for everyone to learn and understand. Keeping your spine flexible and learning to move it correctly is a skill we are not taught at school. In Chi Kung the spine is the core link between heaven and earth. This means it acts like a power rod for the movement of Chi through your centre, flowing from above and below you. Your Chi level is largely to do with how well this connection is established in your system and how well Chi flows.

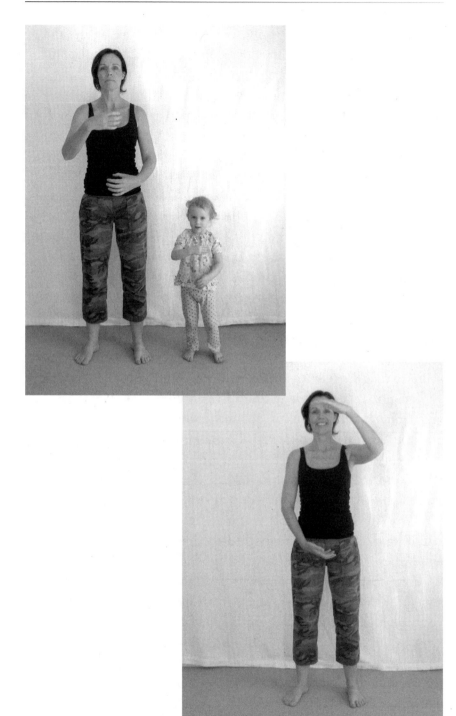

The more connected you are to these ascending and descending natural forces, the more energized you feel. A great way of deepening this connection is to simply get in touch with the energy movements. There are many Chi Kung exercises for this, but the simplest is to mimic these movements. Let your palms lead as you take your hands up from the bottom of your spine at the pelvis to the spine at the top of your neck. Let your hands turn at both ends and move slowly in the opposite direction.

It takes time to attune to these forces and the subtle flows of Chi. Chi Kung is mostly about bringing your mind and body to a heightened state of sensitivity. The best place to start is with increasing your body awareness. Your whole body orientates around the spine, so you will naturally start to notice increasingly more about your spine and its pivotal part in the body. In fact, what is the spine? We use this word a lot, but what exactly is it? Is it the spinal column with all its joints and vertebrae? Is it the ligaments that bind the column together? Is it the multitude of muscles that associate with the spinal column? Is it the ribs which all join into the vertebral column? Is it the spinal cord and spinal nerves that innervate the organs, glands, muscles and bones of the body? Where does the spine end? Is the head part of the spine? Is the brain part of the spinal cord? Is the sacrum part of the spine or part of the pelvis? Is the spine the body? Is the body the spine? Is the spine a connector to creative forces that flow subtly through the body without our being aware of it, sustaining us and keeping us alive? How do we know that this isn't true? Can you feel your nervous impulses moving through your body now? Can you feel the hum of your nervous system, making millions of synaptic connections every second? Most people can't and so they can only believe this to be true from what they read in books. With practice you can increase your body sensitivity so that you are aware of these movements. You enter an exquisite world of connection to your cells and tissues that reveals a new dimension of life and the subtle flow of Chi, and ultimately of you.

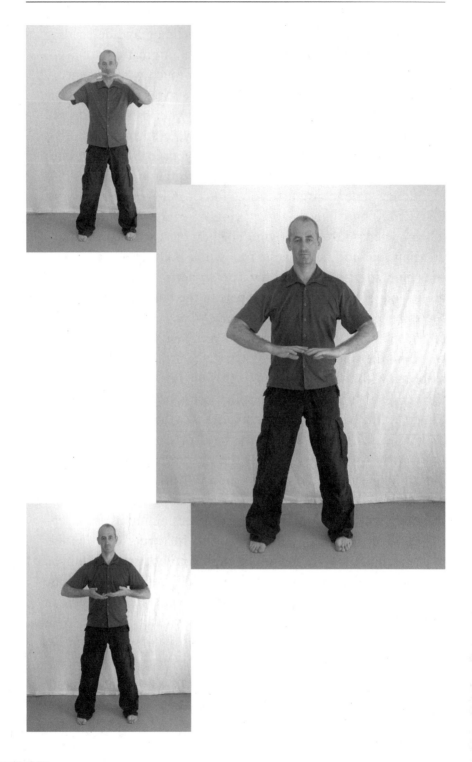

Chapter 2

LISTENING TO YOUR BODY

It's astonishing how we are taught to ignore and override our body messages. This process starts from birth and sometimes before birth. We are not taught to listen and be sensitive, or to rely on our instincts. How wonderful it would be if schools had lessons in being sensitive and in how to listen to your body. What sort of society would that produce? Many people in the world have stopped listening – there have been simply too many messages to discourage listening to their bodies for too long. Reversing that process is no small thing. It takes focus and persistence but, once engaged, this innate wisdom will start to emerge quickly. When you start to hear what your body is telling you, then you can begin to practise intelligent exercise that allows you to provide your body with the right kind of movement it needs for strength and mobility. Not movement you "think" it needs. For most of us the ideas we have about how to exercise derive from the collective construct of fitness. This might be fine for some people, but it ignores individual needs. We are all different, and many people will not respond well to strong exercise. What your body needs is strengthening so that muscles and connective tissues are communicating, connected and "alive". All the exercises in this book will be performed differently by each individual, therefore every movement will be unique to you and to your body. It is important to focus on the intentions behind each exercise and improve the ability to listen to and sense your body's requirements. That means learning not to override them. So the place to start is to find out what's going on in your body.

A well known Chi Kung exercise is called "shaking" and it can take a while to get the hang of it. Shaking is about letting your body go; letting it loosen up. Start by just allowing your body to move into an up/down motion. Stay with this for a while so you can find a rhythm to it. Don't work too hard at it. Notice your spine as you shake. It should be subtly "concertina-ing" along its length. You may find parts of your spine unable to do this, as some areas may be held and unable to move freely. No matter. Just stay with the shaking in a relaxed way, keeping part of your awareness on your spine, and you will notice it starts to loosen up in areas that were initially resistant. As you continue to practise shaking, your spine will gradually lose these areas of tension and you'll be able to move more freely. As a result the rest of your body will loosen too. The spine connects all things, so its health reflects into the rest of the body.

If you've got a tight neck, your arms are probably not going to be too mobile. If you are tight between the shoulder blades you are probably breathing poorly. Shaking first helps dissolve tension patterns in the superficial muscles of the spine such as the trapezius, then it will act on deeper muscles, and eventually on the deepest muscles that link the vertebrae together. This is where a lot of deep-seated tension that might have been stored there for years can exist in you. These muscles are rarely engaged in western-style exercise, where most of the emphasis is on the superficial and intermediate muscle groups. There are thousands of these deep muscles which can be activated through shaking. The state of these muscles has a significant effect on the flow of Chi along the central channels.

Once you've shaken the whole spine for a while, use the shaking to focus into each spinal segment, starting from the bottom of the spine. Do this by taking your attention to this part and

LISTENING TO YOUR BODY

feeling into the bottom of the spine as it meets the sacrum in the pelvis. Shake so that you specifically loosen this part of the spine, then shift to the next higher segment and do the same with that. You can then begin to work up through the length of the spine over a few sessions of shaking. Once you've done this you will know the health of your spine and be able to identify areas that are dense and painful and have poor Chi flow, and areas that are healthy, open and flowing. So spend time shaking into these areas to loosen them up. It might take a while if the tensions have been there for a long time, but persistence will pay off. You will feel like a different human being.

This time, as you shake, listen/feel how your body is as a whole. So widen your attention out from your spine. Again, where are the places that feel good in the shaking? Where are the places that feel as if they are not participating? Take time to notice this. Some places will be obvious. This is a process of self-diagnosis. Once you have mapped this out, you can use an image to facilitate letting go of tensions. Simply imagine the tensions dissolving, melting from solid to fluid. When the body feels more fluid, movement becomes a pleasure and you feel great. Some areas in your body will take some convincing to ease up, so repeating the shaking and dissolving will bring results. The body likes the familiar and responds well to a known movement, and responds even better when this is combined with using an intention such as the intention to dissolve. It is common for there to be one or two dominant places in the body that feel tight and painful.

At first shaking can be awkward and uncomfortable. Most of this is unfamiliarity, as shaking highlights the way the body isn't coordinated or fluid in its movements. One of the key areas that prevents a smooth movement is the groin. In Chi Kung this area is called the "kwa" and is a combination of the hip joint, muscles, ligaments and nerve/blood vessels. It commonly becomes tense and held through poor posture and emotional compression. Shaking into these areas can greatly relieve this tension and allow

Chi to flow more easily between the pelvis and legs. Often the existence of tension here is the cause of why people don't feel grounded or can't make a Chi connection to the earth.

Put the palm of your hand onto this area from the front and the other hand on the back of the pelvis and see if you can shake into the area between your hands. Don't worry about what kind of shaking comes from here, just let your body go into an instinctive movement. This will work into the body tissues and encourage Chi to flow in the area. There is a constant relationship between the physical body and Chi. The two are intertwined, and connecting with both is essential for release. Make sure you always acknowledge the body tissues and the Chi in the body, and in the field around the body. Then you are recognizing the whole expression of the human system, and deeper and quicker changes take place.

Chapter 3

NATURAL ALIGNMENT

We are all subject to gravity, but since we are bipedal and upright we are subject to these forces in a particular way. Our body has to expend a lot of energy trying to find the optimum position for weight to be equally distributed along the length of it – particularly through the spine and pelvis. A large part of the brain is constantly engaged with this specific task. Consider how much less energy you would consume in movement, standing or sitting if you were able to develop the skill to align your joints in a way that optimized your body's posture, minimizing the pressure and strain through the length of it. As a result, your body would be more relaxed and you would achieve a certain equilibrium in your physiology. The consequences of this would certainly be a greater degree of health and you could even extend your life expectancy!

However, what happens if you're not this person and your body, through habit or trauma, is not in perfect alignment? You can imagine the compensations your body would have to make; tension would be part of who you are, and you would get tired just from standing and walking. There would be wear and tear in your joints and you would have to accommodate varying degrees of aches and pains.

What few people really grasp is that you can change these habits. Hardly anyone has perfect alignment and symmetry in their body, but you can optimize and transform your health through some simple exercises. First, find out how your body aligns itself with gravity. The best way to do this is simply to stand for a while, as still and quietly as you can, and observe how your body "stands". It might initially feel strange just to stand still for a while and watch yourself. There might be urges to move, either to walk somewhere or to move a part of the body. Those urges will diminish after standing for a couple of minutes and you will soon be able to observe clearly how your body stands. Here are some key questions to consider:

- How does it feel to stand still?
- Is your body happy to do this or does it feel uncomfortable?
- Is it an effort?
- Does it hurt? / Is it a strain?
- Are there any areas that particularly feel stressed?
- Do any areas feel good?
- What's going on in your spine?

Stay with this exercise for five minutes. Time it. Standing still like this is a Chi Kung practice and, as you can see, it's very revealing. It's also healing. If you stood like this every day for a few days, you would notice that the "standing" becomes easier and there's less resistance in mind and body, creating an automatic strengthening and re-posturing. It's as if the body, given the chance to be with itself in a conscious way, will start to adjust to a more efficient and balanced form. It's a major awakening when you discover this and allow the implications of this knowledge to filter through every aspect of your being.

Given the right set-up, your body will readjust itself. You don't have to do anything. Just stand there. Can you believe it? There's no effort required, you don't need to go to the gym for years and work hard. You just stand every day for five minutes – and you will have more energy, more strength, and you'll minimize all your aches and pains. Give it a try. In reality, we don't ever really stand still in a conscious way. We're always walking and moving, doing things or, if we are standing, our minds are so active we're somewhere else. The task is to stand and be still, with absolute inner awareness of how our body "stands", right now.

It would be useful, after you've finished standing, to spend a few minutes writing down what came to you, especially where it feels good and where it feels uncomfortable or painful. Often it's a case of one side feeling fine while the other side feels strained and uncomfortable. This is fairly common and it's good to write it down, as it will help you describe what is happening in your body. It's a bit like doing a self-assessment, and you'll be impressed by how much detail can come to you.

Helping your body to realign in this way can dramatically increase your sense of well-being and state of health. Experimenting with the way you stand is particularly effective in helping your body to do this.

Mechanically there are some basic facts of life. Here are a few.

- Your spine needs to have its natural curves as well as to be held as vertically as possible.

- Your weight-bearing joints in the pelvis and legs need to be optimally positioned so that weight passes through the centre of the joints.

- Your feet need to take the weight of the body through the heels and forward through the length and width of the feet.

These three points are critical for good posture and good life. Chi Kung focuses a lot of attention on producing these effects.

We'll be looking at a practice to bring all these joints into better alignment. However, before moving on to that, there is something else to consider. What effect will stilling the mind have on posture? As your mind becomes less active and more disposed to being quiet and relaxed, will this affect your body? The answer is that it will, enormously. One of the big drivers behind poor posture is the state of the nervous system. The more stressed you get, the more your posture distorts. If the nervous system is too excited, the body starts to tense up and malfunction, so just by slowing your brain and nervous system activity down you change how your muscles, organs and joints behave. This understanding has enormous implications, just to simply practise being quiet. This practice is in itself a powerful exercise regime. As the mind becomes quieter, the body is more efficient and it starts to be able to form a more direct relationship to Chi, rather than the haphazard one that is the case for most people. Then you start to notice Chi movements in your body all the time and the body becomes suffused with it, leading to more energy, more creativity and a sense of youthfulness. More about this later.

Try this exercise.

Begin by standing in the way you normally do. Let your mind relax. Bring your awareness to your head, and its position at the top of the spine. How does it feel? Let's see how it likes to move. Slowly rotate your head to the left, and then to the right. Which way does it like to go? Position your head so it's in the most comfortable place in one of the rotations.

Then do the same for up-and-down movements. Nod your head forwards and then backwards. Again, which position does your head feel most comfortable in? Place your head there.

Now, let's side-bend the head, both left and right. Which feels better? Place your head in that position, and then re-establish the rotation and nodding positions so you've brought all three together, and end up with a position that is a composite of the three.

Having achieved a comfortable position for your head, move down to the shoulders and do the same thing. Move your right shoulder forward and your left shoulder backwards so you take your whole shoulder girdle into a rotation. Now repeat the opposite way. Which movement is easiest? Bring your shoulders into a position in that plane that makes your body feel most comfortable. Now raise your right shoulder, now raise your left shoulder and arrive at a position that feels most comfortable. Now shift your attention to your pelvis and hips. Shift your right hip out to the right, then your left hip out to your left so you take the pelvis into a sidebend with the spine. Now take the right hip forward and then the left. In both cases find the place of comfort, so that the pelvis is positioned with a sense of ease. Now move your awareness to your feet. Shift your weight towards the balls of the feet, then shift it back towards the heels. Find a place in between the two which feels most balanced and where the body feels like it is doing least work. Once you have worked through these balancing movements let your body stand still and experience the sense of alignment through the length of the body. Notice how Chi moves through your body now. You can do this exercise with much more detail working with each vertebra of the spine and each of the leg joints to allow an even greater optimization of your posture and therefore a greater flow of Chi.

Chapter 4

BREATHE
MORE

B reathing is necessary for life; though you would hardly believe it, as so many people seem to restrict their breath to
shallow arrhythmic motion or to gasping and panting. Your body
will be much more energized with deeper, fuller breaths, and can
be super-energized with a breath that involves the whole body.
Breathing is taking in the environment, taking it deep inside
your body, into your blood. Strange thought, that. It allows the
outside world to be taken into all your cells in fluid form. "As you
breathe, so shall ye reap" – which is not a biblical expression, but
should be. One of the commandments should be "Breathe and
you will be free". Your life depends on your breath.

Physiologically, you are delivering molecules of oxygen to
your cells and expelling carbon dioxide. Poor breath means you
are not creating enough pressure at the surface area of the lungs,
so there's a poor uptake of oxygen. Cells are therefore deprived
of oxygen, and the activity within cells diminishes. Metabolism
slows down, and you become sluggish in mind and body. It also
leads to poor posture. Holding your breath or breathing shal-
lowly means that your body is tense in the chest and shoulders,
and this fixes the spine and allows for little movement in the
upper body. You may have noticed this in yourself when you get
stressed; it's as if you lose your suppleness, and you start to move

in a blocked way. The body is a whole unit, and works best when all the parts of it are moving together. Should one part of the body not move so freely, well, then the rest is affected. You can test this out very simply. Try walking with your jaw clenched. You will quickly notice how strangely you start to walk, and how unbalanced you become.

This next movement is very useful for gradually opening up the chest and creating a stretch along the inside of the arms to the shoulder joints. As you deepen into the stretch, the ribcage opens up and all the muscles at the front of the chest slowly ease, allowing you to breathe more fully. As your body warms up in this exercise you can drop more fully into the stretches, and the spine in the chest starts to bend more powerfully. The trick with this exercise is to take your time with it and work with the body. Listen to your body and don't strain or over-extend in the stretches. Allow your breath to synchronize with the movement so that you inhale as you open up the arms and chest and exhale as you bring your arms down.

Begin with your hands hanging down by the sides of your body and next to the pelvis. Let your wrists be soft, so that you can lead with the wrists as you bring your arms upwards in front of the shoulder joints. At the top of the movement the palms temporarily look forward. Turn the hands ninety degrees and move the hands outwards and widen across the body out to the sides palms looking at each other then looking forward. This whole movement is on the in breath. As you move into the out breath take the hands in the opposite direction, so narrowing into the arms and chest and moving the hands back down to the sides of the pelvis.

Now that your breath is fuller and your chest more supple, try the next exercise. The intention here is to let your breath deepen even further. The image to hold in mind is of bringing your breath down into the body. This will allow your abdomen to soften and take part in breathing so that you start to breathe deeper. Bring your awareness to your breathing for a few breath

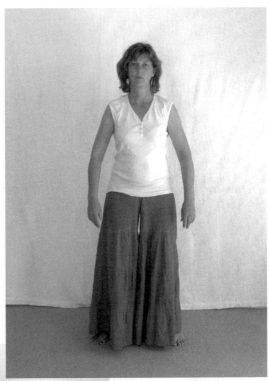

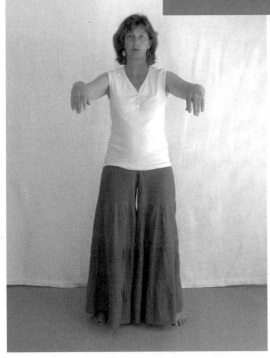

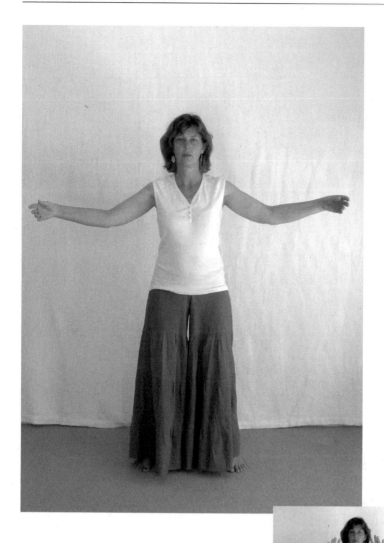

cycles. Bring your hands up high out from your head and as you breathe in, follow the in breath with your hands. So move the hands down toward the chest and then along the front of the body to the pelvis and as you breathe out, take the hands in the opposite direction. As you repeat the exercise, imagine that your breath can move through the whole of your body down to your feet and into the space around you. The hand and arm movements are mimicking this. As you can see, the movement becomes a whole body action. Notice how your body responds to this. There's a subtle energy in the body that can start to flow and it can feel as if you're actually breathing into your feet, into the whole body and the space around you. When this happens, bring the exercise to a close and simply stand still observing your body, noticing how you feel after the two breathing exercises.

BREATHING INTO THE DAN TIEN

The pelvis holds a Chi space, called the Dan Tien, which acts like a reservoir for Chi in the lower body. Dan Tien means "field of bliss". Once your breathing becomes freer and more "whole body" you can start to use your breath to connect with the Dan Tien at the centre of the pelvis. As you practise Chi Kung more often, connecting your Dan Tien with your breath starts to become automatic and natural so that all your movements and your breathing are oriented towards your Dan Tien (more of this in the next chapter). Try placing your hands on your lower abdomen and following your breath into the centre of your pelvis. This is a great way to find the Chi centre of the pelvis and to create an easier energy flow through the Dan Tien.

The classic theory in Chi Kung is that you bring Chi into the body through food and breathing. Your health and vitality are therefore dependent on how well you eat and breathe, along with the quality of the air and food. Poor breathing means you are bringing poor amounts of Chi into your body, so you become

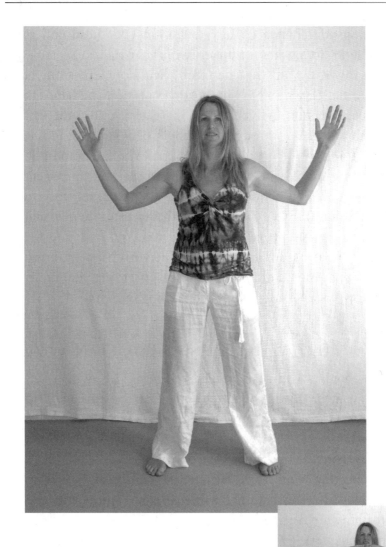

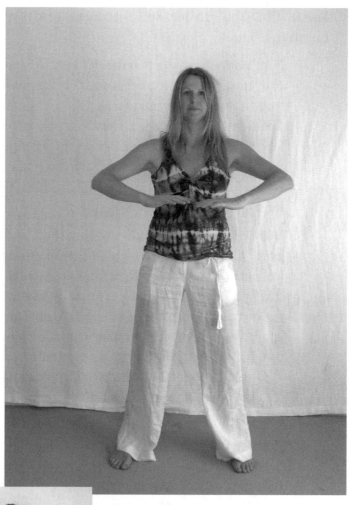

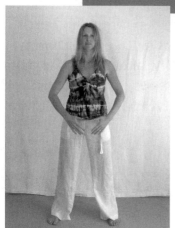

low in Chi. You can increase the intake of Chi through your breath in a number of ways.

- First, notice how you breathe. It's vital to know the state of your breath in order to change it. Try following how you breathe so that you can identify the areas that particularly feel tight or restricted. Often it is part of the breathing mechanism that is the cause. It can be your diaphragm that is tight or it might be the intercostal muscles between some ribs or, again, it might be tension in the shoulders. Find out which of these it might be.

- Use dissolving techniques to bring these areas out of tension. You can imagine that the tense areas are made of ice, and that the ice is thawing out. Mental images have strong effects on the body, especially when you associate the image with a place in the body. Using the breath itself can help dissolve tensions and stagnation by directing the breath into the area. Or simply suggest to your body that it relaxes. If you know what needs to relax, then asking it to relax often has a big effect. You can practise letting go of tension and become good at it.

- Practise taking in more air. You can get your chest to become used to taking deeper breaths by using deep breathing techniques regularly. There are two ways to do this. Have times where you do deep breathing exercises (see below). Maintaining this over a period of time will change the way you breathe. The second way is to practise conscious breathing throughout the day, so that you are watching yourself as you breathe. Using both ways can be even more effective.

- Do specific Chi Kung exercises to increase the flow of Chi. Forms are particular Chi Kung movements and poses that work on different elements, organs, channels or parts of the body. Lung forms will increase the flow along the

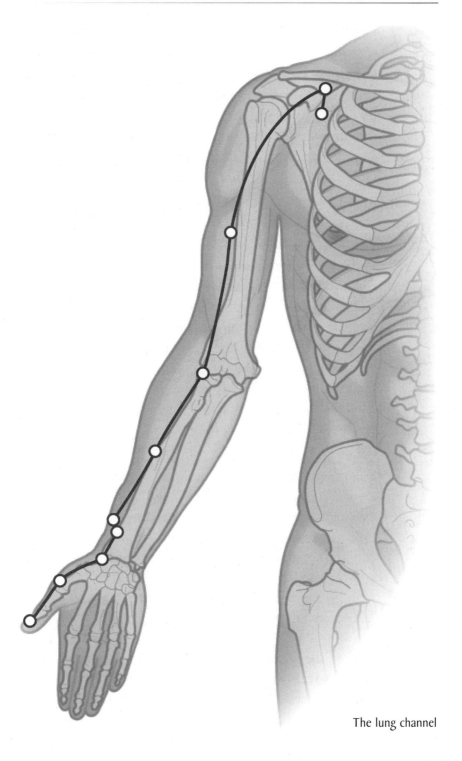

The lung channel

lung channel and in the organ. A particularly good one is to use tapping. Simply tap along the length of the arm using your loose fist following the path of the lung channel as in the image above to the top of the chest then back down again. Repeat this a few times then move to the other arm. Often the channel can get quite hot as it activates the lungs. Once the lungs have been filled with more Chi, your breathing will naturally deepen.

- Another useful method is to connect with the air around you and follow the movement of air into the lungs. As you start to follow this, shift perspective so that you open up to the perception of a much bigger space around you and feel into the subtle qualities of this space. This is the Chi, and you should feel lighter and energized just by coming into contact with it. Your body has a powerful connection to the universal Chi field via your lungs. At a physical level your lungs are moving air in and out, but at a Chi level there's more of an absorption of the Chi, as if there's a natural gradient that makes the Chi gather in the lungs. See what happens as you widen your perception of and relationship to the Chi field around you. Do it slowly.

- Using sounds. Chi Kung designates sounds for various organs and making the "lung sound" can be a powerful way of transforming tension patterns and allowing the breath to deepen. Sounds create a resonant vibrational pattern that directly relates to the function of any particular organ. Bringing a vibrational pattern into relationship with an organ allows it to re-set itself, so to speak, or release any held patterns. The original sound for lungs is a "Shee-aye", but most sounds that are made with the "eee" in them can work well. Take a long, slow breath in and make this sound on a slow exhale. A powerful way to make the sound is to connect with the earth through the feet and allow the sound to resonate through the lungs.

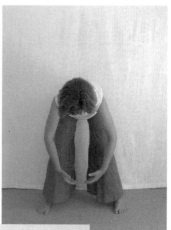

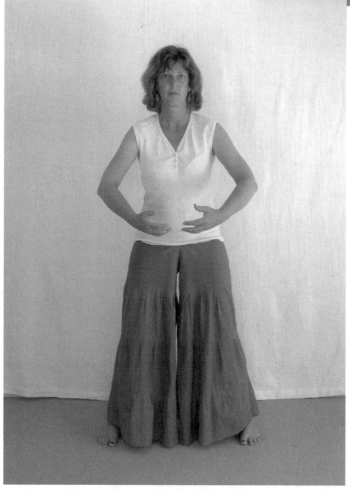

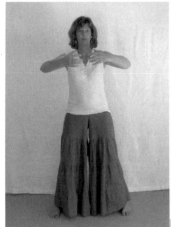

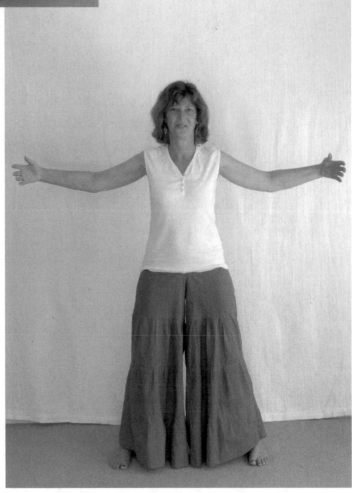

Take a stance that will allow you to use your whole body and feel the support of it. The sequence above shows how the form can be used to create strong Chi effects in the lungs and therefore change your breathing as a result.

- Moving in synchrony with your breath. All Chi Kung forms can be synchronized to your breathing. This combination of movement and breath is "breathtaking" in its internal response, creating a greater Chi effect. It's important to start with the movement to synchronize with your breath and not the other way round. You want to avoid straining or fighting with your breathing. As you continue with the synchronized form there will be a natural lengthening and deepening of your breathing. A great example of this are Chi Kung walks which we will look at in greater detail later.

A simple form for the lungs would be opening the hands and arms from the chest and then gathering the hands back to the same place. As the hands open out you breathe in, and as they come back to face the chest, you breathe out. Practising this as a whole body movement rather than concentrating just on your hands and arms means that Chi throughout the body is accessed while doing the form.

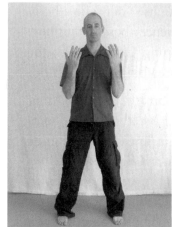

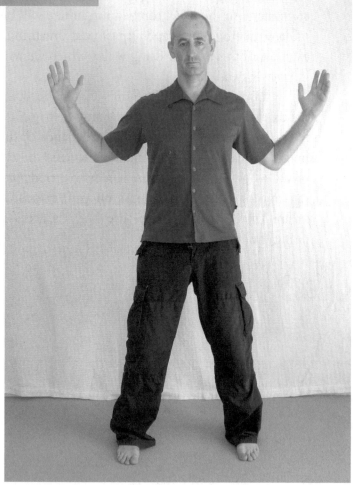

Chapter 5

A NEW
PELVIS

Where is the centre of the body? In relation to gravity and movement the pelvis is a vital place in the body. Mechanically, it translates the weight of the upper body from the torso to the ground. The pelvis is where the legs meet the spine. The legs are there for walking and the spine is there for connecting the torso. If you can truly move from the pelvis then you can move with strength and energy. Many people move from places higher up in the body, as if that's their centre of gravity. Often it's the chest. Watch people as they move; see if you can tell where their centre of gravity is. Unfortunately, for many people the pelvis is a place of tension and poor movement. The hip joints are often held very tightly from muscle tension in the groin, the pelvic floor and the lower back. These places can be some of the tightest places in the body, and are often held unconsciously. There are some simple movements that can free the pelvis from its prison of tension.

This is such a simple movement. Circling the pelvis. However, give it a try and you will see that it's not as easy as it seems. Place your hands on the back and front of the pelvis, make sure your knees are bent, and try to move from a place between your hands. Let the movement be smooth, and as perfect a circle as you can create. As you move in a circle, try to rock the pelvis front to

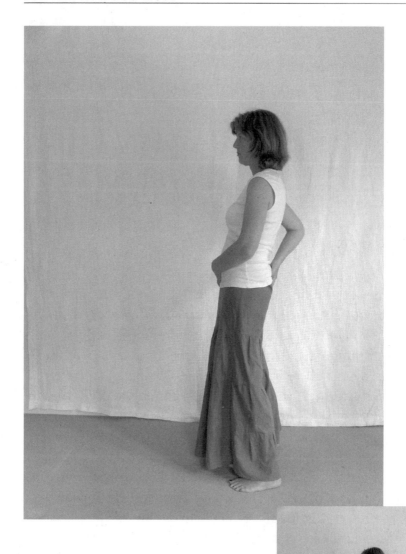

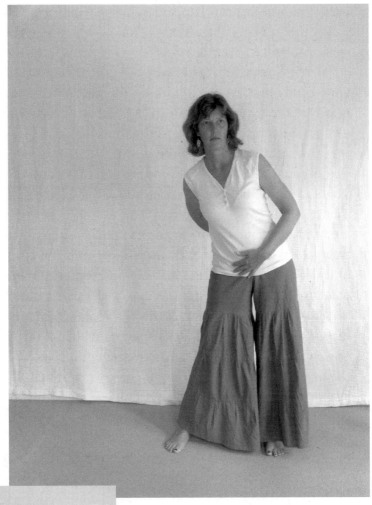

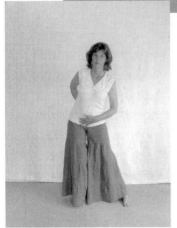

back. You can feel this happening in the hand at the back of the pelvis that touches the sacrum. This will help free some of the tension. Try it in both directions.

Here's a more energetic way to open the pelvis. Take both your hands and let the centre of the palms look towards the centre of the front of the pelvis. Move both hands around until you get a deep sense of connection into the pelvis. The palm of the hand is an important place in Chi Kung as it contains a Chi that is connected to the fire element and the centre of the chest. There are a number of theories about the location of the Dan Tien in the pelvis, but the best way to find it is to explore this area with the palms of the hands. Let the hands move close to the front of the pelvis, and then away more into the space in front of it. Shift the angle of the hands until eventually there's a sense of a significant connection. People feel this in different ways: tingling, flow, magnetic or electrical sensations, increased space/ expansiveness, the mind goes quieter, exhilaration, grounded-ness, a sense your hands can't move, sensations in other parts of the body, wholeness, building of energy in the pelvis. These are just some examples of the many things you might experience in Chi Kung practice.

Stand like this for a few minutes, then let the hands open out to the sides of the pelvis, fingers looking down. Hold that for a minute and notice what happens. Then bring the hands back in to the centre slowly, then repeat the movement, moving at a constant slow speed, opening out to the sides and gathering back to look at the centre of the pelvis. As you continue there should be an increased sense of flow and connection in and around the pelvis, which spreads to the rest of the body over time. Spend ten minutes doing this and then notice how you are for the next few hours. Particularly, how you walk, how you perceive things around you, what state your mind enters, your energy levels, how you relate to others. Over time this practice will have profound effects. The fundamental change will be that it makes you feel more centred in body and mind. Suddenly you are moving from

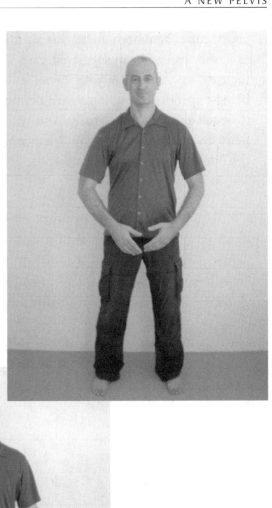

your centre. The body loves this, as it can move more efficiently as a unit instead of in separated parts. Your physical energy will increase as you are moving more efficiently, so less energy is being expended. Your mind will be less frenetic, it will be easier to focus and to think clearly. You will have a stronger sense of body awareness and along with this a sense of Chi in and around the body.

Chapter 6

KNOW
YOUR FEET

O ur feet can seem a long way from our intellect and unless there is pain or discomfort, we hardly pay them any attention. The feet have an amazing structure. At first it might seem a bit ungainly, but as you take a closer look you will notice that feet take all the body's weight and distribute it, spreading it into the ground, as well as having an elastic tension along their full length that acts as a "spring system" to allow for an agile response.

If the feet are unable to express their natural movement, it's usually a reflection of enormous tension. The main cause of this is how the joints in the legs are aligned and, in turn, how the joints of the lower spine entering the pelvis are aligned.

Alignment here is critical for allowing the body's weight to spread evenly through the pelvis and down the legs. Our posture is everything. We hold ourselves in all kinds of strange shapes. A very common example is tilting the pelvis and locking the legs whereby we end up with painful joints and imbalanced muscle tone. Some muscles will over-compensate for those that have become lax and do not support the joints. Over time this results in strain through the lower joints of the body, and tension in the feet as they try to cope with the issues above them. Try getting a foot massage or reflexology and notice how much pain and discomfort there can be in your feet.

A lot of emphasis is given to making the feet healthier in Chi Kung. There are seventy-six million nerve endings in the soles of the feet, which is twice the number in the hands! So it shows how sensitive they are, and how much we blot them out of our daily consciousness. We are so much more oriented to our hands. Overall, we perceive our world mostly through our hands, face, eyes, ears, mouth and nose. That means that there's a whole lot of information from the rest of our body we're not listening to, and the feet are no different. The important thing is to relax your feet. Creating an alignment of joints and posture will allow the body to deal more efficiently with standing and walking. Spending time becoming more aware of your feet can transform your life.

There is a way to become sustained by Chi through the connection of your feet and that is the wisdom of Chi Kung. It's crucial to make a relationship with the centre of your feet. In Chi Kung this place is called "bubbling spring" and is located just behind the balls of the feet, in line with the third toe and the heel. This is an important gateway for the flow of Chi into the body. Opening up to this creates a deeply significant relationship that anyone can have with the earth. Bringing your awareness into this area will allow you to develop a connection that brings about Chi flow, from the earth, through the feet and into the whole body, reviving you and making you light.

LET THE GROUND SUPPORT YOU

Standing comfortably, make sure your knees are not locked. Let your feet be parallel and hip-width apart, and let your arms hang loosely by your sides. Notice how you feel now. Then let your head relax. Do that by consciously becoming aware of and easing up any tensions. Your body will respond to this. Next let your shoulders and neck support your head so that your head can drop into the shoulders. Then bring your awareness to your shoulders. Let tensions dissolve. Then let your shoulders drop downwards and let them be supported by your chest. Let the tensions in your chest dissolve, and let it be held by the spine and the abdomen. Let your abdomen relax and let it be supported by your pelvis. Let the pelvis relax and be supported by the legs. Let your legs relax and be supported by the feet. Let your feet relax and be supported by the ground. Now let your whole body relax into the ground. Let the ground support you. Now, how does your body feel?

Bubbling spring

Now that your weight is more fully in your feet, bring your awareness to the centres of your soles. Let your awareness rest lightly here. Stay like this for a couple of minutes, then use the image of a bubbling spring. Imagine a natural flow of water coming into the feet from the earth through this place. Stay with the image. After a minute, open up to the flow coming up into the body, and notice where it goes. What places in your body respond to the flow of Chi? Let's try to magnify this by placing your hands in front of your pelvis, palms down. Move your hands so that the centres of your palms look at the centres of your feet. This should intensify the Chi flow. Stay like that for a couple of minutes, and then let your whole posture and the image dissolve.

Bubbling spring is at the first point on the kidney channel and is considered to be vital to the healthy flow of Chi in the lower body. When we allow it, Chi will flow naturally up the body from the earth and will act like a spring, bringing new life to the body. When you learn to access this, it will enable you to recharge quickly and to improve your health. At a deeper level it brings Chi not just into the kidney organs, but also into the central channels.

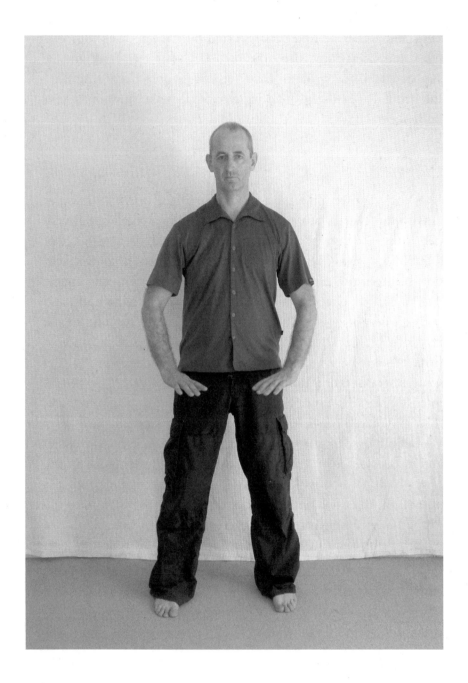

CONNECTING THE HANDS AND FEET

There are some relationships in the body that are particularly profound and resonant. The way the hands and feet connect with each other is one of the body's great phenomena. In traditional Chi Kung this is thought of as uniting fire and water. Just bringing the hands and feet into a connection will instigate a balancing of the fire and water elements in the body/Chi system. The water is cooling, and its orientation is downwards; whereas fire is heating, and its action is upwards and outwards. So relating the hands with the feet instigates a meeting and balancing of these two great forces.

THE FEET AND THE PELVIS

The centre of the foot is a wonderful place to align the centre of the pelvis with, as this creates a natural flow from the earth through each foot, up the legs and into the Dan Tien. You can try this out in a simple way by rocking back and forth from a standing position. Where is the place that feels most balanced, so that your weight is being spread evenly across the full length of the feet?

Try also to let your weight spread evenly across both feet. Find the bubbling spring and see if that changes anything. Now bring your awareness to the Dan Tien at the centre of the pelvis and observe how Chi flows from the feet to the pelvis and how your posture changes. Stay with it for a while, then start shifting your weight from one leg to the other. Let it be a gradual shift so that you can follow how your body does this with attention. It feels as if the Dan Tien is moving directly over each bubbling spring, and there's suddenly a deeper connection. Allow the movement to be smooth as your centre of gravity moves from left to right. Try altering your foot positions slightly and see if that makes a difference in the smooth shifting of weight. This is a great exercise for increasing the flow of Chi into the legs and encouraging the natural flow of Chi from the earth into the body. Once you have established this understanding and relationship, the Chi flow will enliven you constantly.

Chapter 7

MOVING IN THREE DIMENSTIONS

In this chapter we are going to discuss our understanding of our internal environment in relationship to our exterior environment. Most of us operate in the world in what could be referred to as a two-dimensional experience, i.e. we are mostly not aware of our internal volume and how that relates to the space around us. A world exists where we can relate to all aspects of our environment, that includes our internal volume in connection to our exterior world and lets us become three-dimensional creatures. Let's explore this concept.

When you are thinking a lot, you shift into an internal reverie which, over time, leads to a state where you primarily reside in your thoughts and your intellectual functioning. This draws you away from your body awareness so that your movements are dimly registered. It can feel as if you are operating on automatic pilot. You walk down the road, you catch a bus, you walk through the park, yet you are so entrenched in your own thinking process that you are only partially aware of your body movements and coordination. You have a reduced experience of body sensation, kinaesthetic movement, awareness of what is around you and energetic connection to your surroundings. If you had to stop for a moment and consider your limbs, head and torso, and had to turn all the way around, you might recognize that you are moving in the whole space surrounding you. It's really easy to forget this, as we tend to walk forwards only, and therefore focus and orientate ourselves directly to the things in front of us. However, there actually is a whole space either side of you, behind you, above and below you. Do you walk and consider this experience as three-dimensional motion or do you simply keep walking forwards, lost in your internal mental distractions?

Being completely distracted can, at its worst state, make you feel as if you are a ghost in a machine – simply running on auto-pilot and only engaging with the external world from a mental perspective, for brief spells at a time, before sinking back into reverie. This state can sometimes be a highly creative space or it can be a foggy experience, but in either case it's a shift away from body sensations. Is that a problem? It seems most people operate this way in the world, but what are the consequences?

One could argue that disconnection from the exterior world is a self-preserving, filtering technique, designed to keep us safe. It would be equally fair to say that maybe we wouldn't need to filter out the world if we weren't already so over-stimulated internally. However, what's important to recognize is that what this behaviour is actually doing is shutting down (or out) the natural order of things, i.e. the equal exchange of energy between one's own health and vitality and that of the greater sphere of the environment. In nature, the two are never separate. The more one shuts out or disconnects from the world, the less one can receive any positive influence of any form.

It is actually possible to remain utterly connected to all things around you and still filter out what you choose not to deal with. This would be a higher mechanism of health at work, for conscious choice is involved as opposed to an automatic shut-down (primitive response). Being sensitive to one's internal framework as well as having a strong connection to the external forces at play and using them creates a highly functioning and vital human. In reality, it means that this sort of an individual is functioning at a level where they have a very clear indication of who they are, where they are, what they are doing, what their capacity for health is, and therefore what right decisions to make. Life takes on a very different sort of existence.

In Chi Kung there is an emphasis on both the internal and external Chi flow. Equal importance is given to both. The idea is that there is an external field that emanates out from the body in all directions. What this effectively means is that you come out of yourself and form a relationship with the world around you. This affects you at every level, but practically it means you move with an awareness of your internal body sense as well as the space around you. Suddenly, this can mean you walk and stand in a bigger context. It means that a new balance has to be created within this larger context. Being more aware of your surroundings allows you to be more open to Chi, and this will help you steady yourself in the world. This is a far cry from feeling insular or unsupported.

Here's an exercise for creating a state of balanced awareness, connecting internal and external Chi fields and taking Chi flow to a new level.

Sitting still comfortably, allow yourself to settle and relax. Notice your breathing, notice body sensation. Become aware of movement in the body, as well as stillness. Notice how the body structures organize themselves around your central axis (spine and head). Feel your body as a three-dimensional form, feeling front to back, top to bottom and side to side. Notice how your body occupies space. Can you get a sense of Chi in your body? What is its quality and movement?

Staying with the sense of internal space, become aware of the external space around you. Enter into the world of the senses by tuning into your hearing. And then into your sense of smell. Slowly open your eyes and orient to visual sensation. Experience these senses whilst remaining in contact with your internal space/sensations. What's the Chi like in the external field? How does it feel different from the internal one?

Try to find a state of balanced attention between external sensory experience and internal Chi/space/body-sensation. There will be an interface where your attention can be inclusive of both fields and feels at ease. This is a powerful place that will change from moment to moment, try to follow it so that you stay with the state of balance. Notice what changes occur in your body, mind and consciousness during and after the practice.

Becoming familiar and established in this state will help you keep calm and centred. It will also help you move in a three-dimensional way. Walk with your awareness, not only ahead of you, but surrounding you. Essentially, you are forming a relationship with your Chi field, which is an emanation of organs and energy centres within your body. All energy fields meet in the Dan Tien, at the centre of the pelvis, so if you can relate the external Chi field to your Dan Tien, then you are able to harness all of your Chi. Here's a simple walk that moves from the Dan Tien. This will help you get in contact with the external field and change your awareness to a three-dimensional perception.

Stand with your weight resting in both legs. Place your hands in front of your pelvis, your palms looking at the centre of the pelvis. Move the hands slightly up and down, side to side, closer and further away until you have a sense of connection between your hands and your Dan Tien. Spread your body weight across your feet, and find "bubbling spring". Staying with all these connections, shift part of your awareness so that you can experience the space in front of you, then to the sides, then behind you. Find that place of balanced awareness between all these places. Spend a few minutes doing this. Then take your hands and turn them so the palms look forwards, moving them out to the sides of your pelvis with fingertips pointing down towards the ground. Then bring them back again so that your palms face the centre of the pelvis. Stay with this movement form for a while. (This exercise was explored in more detail in Chapter 5.) The form should help you deepen your state of balanced awareness. The focus of the movement is shifting between the Dan Tien and the space around

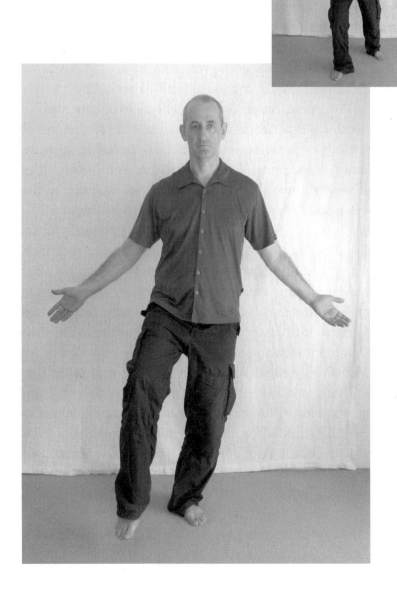

you. Continue this until you have established this relationship, and then move into a slow walk. Start the walk by first shifting your weight into your left leg, then lift the right leg off the floor, place your right heel onto the floor first, slowly pressing your weight into your heel first and then towards your toe. As you do this open the hands out from the pelvis to allow the leg to rise, then, as you step and shift your weight onto the new (left) leg, gather your hands back to the centre of the pelvis. Get used to this movement first, then try to re-establish the state of balanced awareness of yourself and the space around you. This will help you to move through space with greater sensitivity.

We can revisit the walk and look at the details of how to walk from a Chi Kung perspective. But first, let's try to deepen into the three-dimensional experience. Obviously you can't see behind or above you easily or without considerable movement, but you are able to "sense" these places. The "yin" side of your hands, your palms, are very sensitive, and create a powerful intention to the Chi field. Basically, wherever you point your hands there will be a response. You can test this. Stand still and bring your hands to the sides of your pelvis and then turn the palms so they look behind you. Open up to the Chi field behind you. Notice what that feels like – there is a particular quality to it. Then shift the orientation of your palms to the front. Do the same again. Then move the palms so that they look outwards to the sides, then turn them so they look up and, finally, so they look down. All of these fields have a different Chi quality. Now let's go back to the state of "balanced awareness" exercise on page 65 and bring your palms to point at the pelvis. This time, though, connect to each of the spaces around you that you explored with your palm positions. This should give you much more detail about your awareness state. Now shift into the walk and see how that feels.

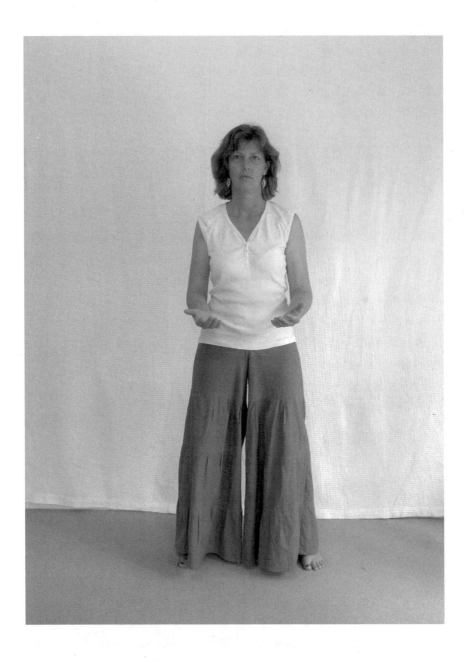

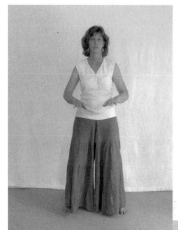

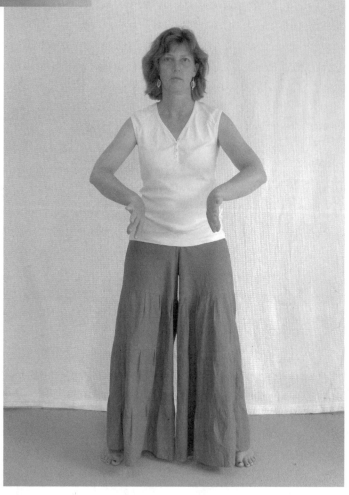

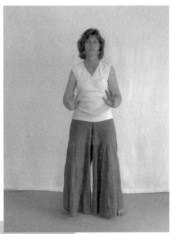

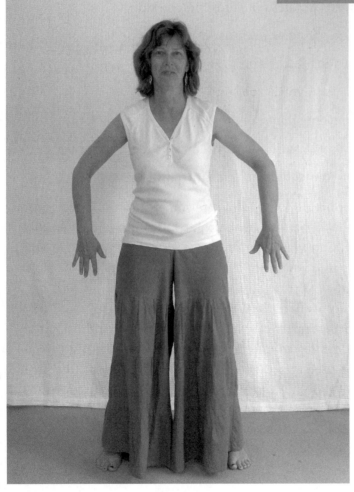

WALKING CHI KUNG STYLE

Walking is something we all do, but when was the last time you noticed exactly how you walk? You might be surprised at what you discover. The next time you walk down the road, watch yourself in a witness-like way. Here are some of the common habits you might notice:

- more weight into one leg

- more power from one leg

- more pressure in your heels or in the balls of your feet

- leg opens (rotates outwards) on one side

- leg closes (rotates inwards) on one side

- knees don't flex much

- tightness in your groin

- pain in some joints

- one side of your body turns towards the front or back

- one of your shoulders leans forward.

What are your hands doing? How are you breathing? Is there tension in your lower back? How much are your abdominal muscles contributing? Can you identify the pace of your walk? Do you feel as if you are running or that you are going too slow? How you walk is how you are. Slow it down and you can work it out. The elements of walking in Chi Kung involve: letting your body weight be borne equally by each leg; getting used to shifting the weight from one leg to another; getting used to sinking as you walk; getting used to raising the leg from the "kwa" (the area of the groin); smooth transition of your weight moving forward from the Dan Tien in the step. The step is everything and can only be worked with by slowing it down. So slow it down.

The first step is to find out what you are doing when you stand. We will go into this in more detail in the next chapter.

Find a space in your room and just stand there in your normal way. Don't do anything different. Where is the upper body weight going? Are you leaning in any direction? Are you really on both feet?

Take a different stance now. Bring both feet parallel and have them hip-width apart, with the outside of the feet in line with the outside of the hips. Bring your awareness to the Dan Tien. Invite your upper body weight to sink through it and move down the legs equally. Then slowly let your Dan Tien shift to the left so that most of the weight travels down the left leg, then shift back to equal weight through both legs, then shift right, weight pressing mostly down the right leg. This can feel like each leg becomes full and then empty.

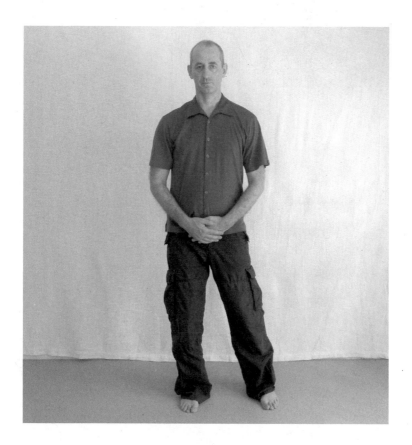

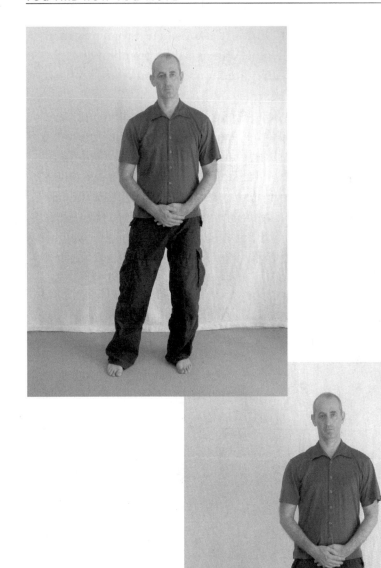

There are hundreds of walking forms, ranging from animal walks, to organ walks, to meridian walks, to elemental walks – all very exciting and inspiring and too many to cover in this book. Let's look at Cloud Walking. The idea behind this is to walk with such lightness and sensitivity that you could walk on a cloud and not fall through it. Placing each foot with a delicate, conscious lightness of step, bringing a state of heightened body awareness that creates a deep connection to your Chi. In the walk there is a synchrony between the hands and feet that produces a strong movement of Chi through the body.

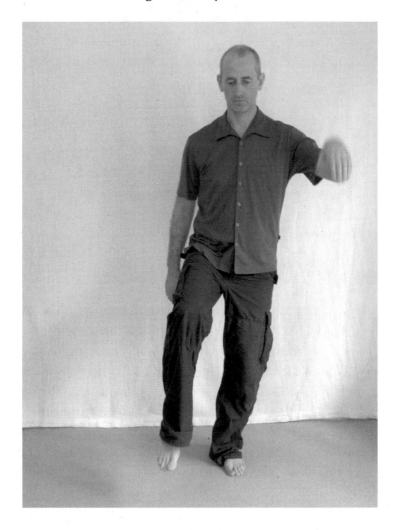

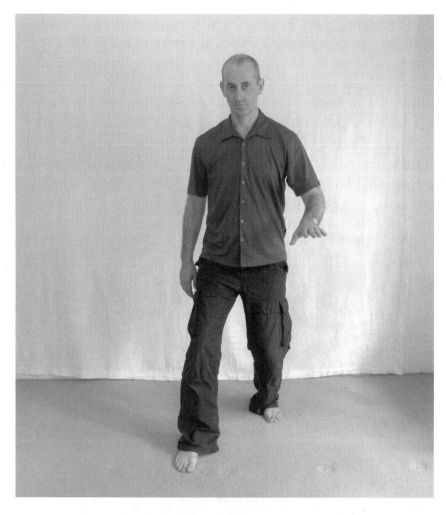

You can see that the walk has an emphasis downwards. The hands become almost like feet, helping to cushion the movements. For you to become accomplished with the walk, there needs to be a connection into the Dan Tien, and a diagonal synchrony between the arms and legs, so that as you raise a leg, the arm on the opposite side is also rising, as if the two are entwined and neither can move without the other. Such cross-hatch movements encourage the brain to be more balanced and mimic many of the nervous impulses that flow from one hemisphere to the opposite side of the body.

The walk can also be done in reverse, which is challenging, but has a remarkable effect in increasing your spatial awareness. The walk is exactly the same, except you are stepping backwards rather than forwards. So rather than placing your heel down first, place the ball of your foot down first, and make sure you don't step too far back. The hand then has more of an emphasis on creating balance. It becomes more of a stabilizer than when you are moving forwards, and there is an even stronger need and emphasis to connect downwards. The centre of the movement shifts from the Dan Tien to a place on the spine behind the umbilicus. This is called the "Gate of Vitality" and is sometimes thought of as the rear Dan Tien. Imagine you have a set of eyes at this place on your spine, so it's as if you feel/see backwards from here. This intention starts to activate this gateway and the walk allows a freeing up and increase of Chi in and around the area.

Chapter 8

THE ART OF
STANDING STILL

It's amazing how standing still is something we do only when we have to: on a crowded bus, train, tube, or in a queue or waiting room, for example. Given the option, most people would prefer to sit down, or walk. People aren't happy standing and quickly become tired and irritable. Why is that? You would expect walking to be more tiring, as it expends much more energy. Few people can stand with ease. When you stand with poise, there is an efficiency in energy expenditure. However, most people cannot stand with poise, so as a result their body consumes even more energy than in walking, trying to compensate for poor posture and distortions in body alignment. People either lock their knees or tilt their pelvis or place their feet at odd angles. This reveals a weakness and lack of strength, plus it indicates how someone is trying to disconnect. In Chi Kung this upright standing posture is called "Wu Chi posture" and is a core practice. It connects you to heaven and earth and opens up a flow of Chi along your central channels, changing your state of consciousness and ultimately bringing you into a relationship with the Tao. "Wu Chi" means "empty energy" and is the ultimate state in Chi Kung. Practise this posture and it will bring you into a strong Chi flow throughout your body and create a vibration that can feel emancipating and peaceful. This state is beyond thought. Your thinking reduces as

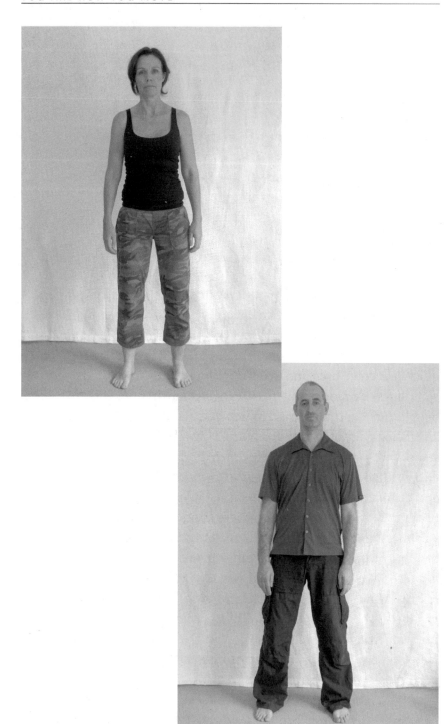

you drop deeper into it, until eventually it stops. Your mind is then free of thoughts and in this state of quiescence you become clear and aware, your body deeply relaxes, and you enter into a fuller relationship with your Chi field and the universal. This feels both centring and expansive. There is a strong infusion of Chi, so you feel highly energized and replenished. A strong Wu Chi connection can feel as if you've had a wonderful deep sleep. Your cells are happy, and there's a feeling of alignment with the natural order of things. This is a movement towards being aligned with the Tao – a concept found in Chinese philosophy that translates as "way" or "path". The Tao signifies the fundamental or true nature of the world as a living, holistic force that is beyond form. The more you bring this into your daily life, the more you will operate with the flow of life. There is no need to buckle from the pressures of life, and take up distorted positions, when you begin to recognize the wisdom and support in the Tao, and the deep satisfaction and replenishment this brings.

BEING CONNECTED IN THE BODY

The trick to attaining a "Wu Chi" state is to bring the whole body into a state of connection with itself and then with the Chi field. There is a belief that you need to practise Chi Kung for twenty years before attaining this, but here's the quick way to get there:

Even if you haven't done this before, you will still experience some aspect of this state; it's just a matter of degree. Stand with feet hip-width apart, feet parallel. Bring your awareness to your Dan Tien and to "bubbling springs" in the centre of your feet. Let all your weight drop into your feet. Slightly tuck your sacrum, so that the pelvis rotates and your lower back lengthens. Tuck your chin towards your neck, so that your spine lengthens. Let your arms go heavy and relax your abdominal wall. Finally let your whole body sink. Bring your attention to the earth below your feet and open "bubbling springs" to the natural Chi flow that moves upwards from the earth. This should be energizing and make you feel buoyant. Now bring your awareness to the space above your head and open up the crown of the head to the natural Chi movement here. The Chi flows downwards and should also feel energizing. This is heaven's force. Now just relax and watch how heaven and earth interact in your body. This is the start of the Wu Chi state. After practising it for some time, these forces harmonize and balance out and then you start to connect with the Tao. The awareness then is of feeling connected, beyond the body, to a universal relationship and a strong sensation of presence. The mind becomes very still and you enter a creative space. This state is the essence of Chi Kung. It's what practitioners are seeking. When you can establish it well, it is with you in all Chi Kung forms, whether standing still or walking.

You can understand why the experience of these dynamic forces has so many greater implications for our health than work on any machine down at the gym will ever achieve.

STANDING FORMS

Chi Kung has taken standing meditations to the level of an art.

There are an infinite number of standing forms in Chi Kung. Each form has its own unique connection to Chi. For instance, if you stand with your hands in front of your chest, this will produce a different effect from putting your hands in front of your pelvis or in front of your head. Try it. It's fascinating how the different cavities of the body create different Chi qualities. In Taoist alchemy these cavities are associated with different Chi. Each Chi is necessary for life and Chi Kung practice aims to bring these three cavities (head, chest, pelvis) into harmony. Bring your hands in front of your chest and point the centres of the palms to the centre of the chest. Let your hands come close and move away from the chest. Find the place where you get the strongest Chi connection. Let your weight drop into the centres of the feet, be a little flexed in your knees, and play around with tucking in your sacrum. The aim is to maximize Chi flow. This can feel like a streaming of energy within you; your mind becomes quiet, your breathing deepens, and there is commonly a sense of expansiveness into the space around you and a sense of your internal body cavities becoming larger and more three dimensional.

Now bring your hands down towards the pelvis and do the same thing here. Palms of the hands point towards the centre of the pelvis. Maximize the effect through adjusting your posture. As you practise you will become more and more sensitive to the adjustments so that it's second nature, and you will notice the Chi effects become stronger and more systemic. Does the Chi quality at the pelvis feel different from that at the chest?

Now bring your hands up in front of the head, point the palms at the centre of the forehead. This stance is trickier, but you can still find a place of comfort and connection if you vary the width of your leg stance and how much you flex your knees, and look for the deepest connection. The Chi in the head is different.

Determine which Chi was the strongest and which was the weakest. For the weakest, keep up the stances and use movement forms to create a flow. With practice the three fields will equalize.

What's interesting is the fact that if your intention is to find the deepest and strongest flow of Chi in the standing postures, you will almost certainly be in classically prescribed Chi Kung stances. These are usually: feet either hip-width or wider apart, kneecaps looking down at the centre of the feet, soft in the "kwa" (the groin area), tucked at the sacrum, soft in the abdomen, tucked at "jade pillow" (top of the spine), soft focus with the eyes open, looking down from the horizontal, dropped shoulder blades.

YIN AND YANG FORMS

With Chi Kung practice your intention is to bring about equality of yin and yang so that you can go behind them to the Tai Chi state. This means you will drop into Wu Chi more easily and deeply. Time slows down and eventually you feel beyond time.

Standing in Wu Chi is standing in the eternal, and time can pass effortlessly. Your body is transformed to the insubstantial force of the Wu Chi state, and you are no longer bound to the physical. In this state you begin to move with the Tao; the force of life is your guide. Your instincts are brought into synchrony with this force. Your mind is then quite different. You are residing in a place behind thoughts, a place where thoughts come from, and increasingly there is a stillness in your mind, so that your mind is mostly oriented towards this, and thoughts are a small part of it.

ORGAN POSTURES

Each organ has its own set of standing postures which are designed to access the Chi system associated with it, and they encourage a particular movement of Chi. Intention is everything in the static postures, and the focus of the mind will create an opening for movement of Chi. For instance, there is a standing pose that creates a flux along the pericardium channel. The "Lao Gong" points, located at the centre of the palms, are points on the pericardium channel, and by bringing them close together in front of the centre of the chest you will create a surge of Chi flow along the length of the channel. You can follow this channel, which runs from the second finger, along the length of the inside of the arms onto the side of the chest, then makes an internal link to the pericardium, which is the membranous tissue surrounding the heart. In Traditional Chinese Medicine this is often referred to as the heart protector.

The heart is such a vital organ that it has an additional set of organs associated with it. Try turning the hands now so that the centres of the palms look inwards. The hands have moved only a few inches and there is quite a different Chi effect. Chi is now oriented much more around the centre of the chest and moves internally within the chest, rather than just around the channel. Now turn the hands so that the palms look out from the chest. That should feel quite different again, and you are now

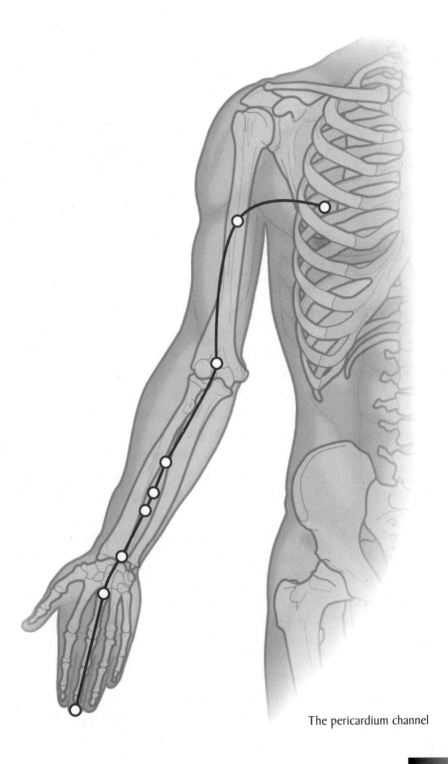

The pericardium channel

connecting to the Chi field in front of you, which has strong associations to the heart, amongst other things. The effect here is to encourage your awareness to move out. Now turn the hands again, but this time with the palms facing downwards. Place one hand on top of the other (it doesn't matter which) and visualize a wooden staff touching the floor between your feet and connecting at the top with the centre of your palm, so that you can lean your weight into it and sink. This posture is called "resting the heart", but it could just as easily be called "earthing the heart", as it does both.

CHI FIELDS

Emanating from the body in all directions is a Chi field. In the Chi Kung paradigm, the body, Chi, mind and emotions are co-existent, not separate. When you start to practise Chi Kung regularly, the external fields start to become very real and present for you. Often one of the effects of Chi Kung is to feel expanded beyond the body. This is the feeling of coming into your Chi fields. How big are these fields? The stronger and healthier you are, the more powerful their emanations. The immediate field is "Wei Chi". This is associated with the skin and the lungs, and acts as immune protection. Further out from the Wei Chi field are the organ fields which, when fully developed, can be extensive, the largest being the yin organs. The heart is felt outwards from the chest, the kidneys out from the lower back, the liver and spleen from the centre-front of the torso, and the lung fields are out laterally and behind the chest. When you become Chi sensitive you can feel these fields and how far they extend. Deeper and more extensive than these are the central channels. The "microcosmic orbit" field can be very extensive and often feels as if it fills the room. The "Chong Mai" field is the biggest of all and can often feel as if it radiates out of the room you are in. This is the channel with most connection to the universal field, which is the natural energy expression within the world around us which our Chi system is always interacting with. (On Chi, see also Chapter 10: "Chi Flow".)

HEAVEN AND EARTH

At the core of all Chi Kung practice is an orientation to the formative energies of heaven and earth. Earth force is a soft rising energy that is often said to turn clockwise as you look down the body. Heaven's force moves in the opposite direction, from above to below, and turns anti-clockwise. Cultivation of these forces and creating a balanced state between them is an ultimate goal in practice. Often we will have a strong preference for one of them. You can test this out for yourself.

Stand somewhere quiet, bring your hands to the umbilical level in the body and turn your hands palms down towards the ground. Stay in this posture for a couple of minutes and notice the effect it has on you. Now turn your hands over, so that your palms look upwards, and stay like this for a couple of minutes. Which direction did you respond to more? Now try the same posture but this time take the hands as far apart as possible so that one hand is below the pelvis with the palm looking down and the other is above the head with the palm looking up. Sometimes when you connect with one of the forces, there may be no response from the other or you might experience strange sensations. This is normally an indication there is a poor expression of this force in your system. Practising these two standing forms will help to transform this and balance the two forces. Practising the movement form that encourages Chi to rise and fall, plus the longitudinal circuits described in Chapter 10, will also help.

INCREASING EARTH

The most common dysfunction in our systems is a poor relationship to the earth force. Many of us are ungrounded and one of the cornerstones of Chi Kung practice is to establish a better

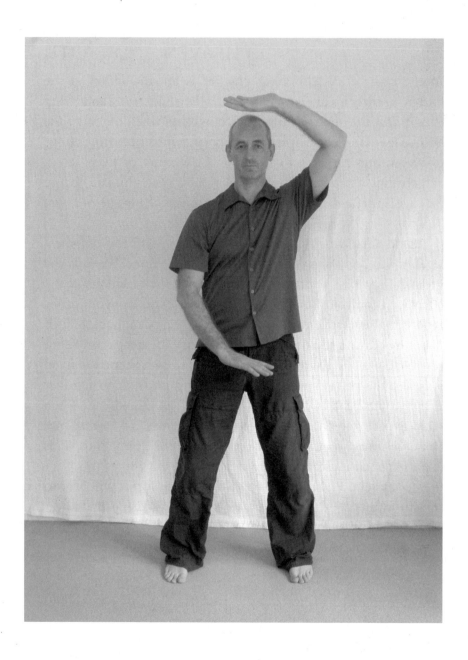

connection with the earth. There are two ways to approach this. One is to work with your preferred force, but keep refining it. In other words, the more fully heaven's force might flow, the more earth's force will be stimulated. The second way is to practise an ancient standing form called "holding the rice sack" and this is a clever form for helping your system connect to earth while staying in contact with heaven. Bring your arms into a right angle at your elbows and turn your palms to look upwards. Imagine you are holding a sack of rice across your forearms. Introducing the image of the rice sack should make the Chi descend, so that you strengthen heaven's force. If you stay with this long enough, say five minutes, you will notice in time that this stimulates a counter-flow upwards.

Alternatively, you can directly encourage the earth flow. This time stand with your palms looking down and use the image of a rising air current, as if you are in an airshaft. Let the movement of air be slow, as too fast will make you feel disoriented. Imagine a slow upward movement like a thermal. Again, see if you are able to experience the counter-flow that might be stimulated.

Chapter 9

OPENING
YOUR JOINTS

O f all the parts of the body, the joints are the most important. This understanding is integral to Chi Kung, and it is often said that "you are as old as your joints". Practitioners of Chi Kung move like water. Their actions are smooth and fluid-like. This stems from suppleness and strength in the joints. It also means that arthritis and other joint degenerative diseases can be avoided. The important thing is to combine the qualities of strength and suppleness. Western exercise can often be too strong for the joints, and they lose their suppleness. Healthy joints are like reservoirs of Chi, full of vitality, so that Chi can easily flow through them. When joints become dense and immobile, Chi can't pass through them easily and this leads to the body becoming fragmented. Chi is less accessible and the body feels fatigued and heavy. This is why people so often feel languid, uninspired and without focus or direction. Working on the joints frees up the restrictions to flow, and the body becomes whole again. Considering how many joints the spine has, working with them and freeing them up will have a big impact. The arms and legs are key areas for the flow of Chi, and the joints in the limbs need constant attention to remain expansive. Let's look at them more closely.

WRISTS AND ANKLES

These joints are so often tight and immobile because people hold them in one position for long periods of time, and rarely flex or extend them. Computer keyboards have a bad effect on the wrists. The hand can hold many tensions that just don't get released and so become set in a pattern for years. Try circling the wrists.

This is such a simple exercise, but the benefits are remarkable. You will be surprised what happens in other parts of your body when the wrists start to relax and expand. In Chi Kung the connection to the centre of the hands is crucial, and any damming up of Chi here will affect the whole system dramatically. Try circling the wrists and the ankles every day for a week, just for a few minutes, and notice the difference. The ankle joints are so often forgotten and can cut off Chi flow from the earth into the body, and vice versa.

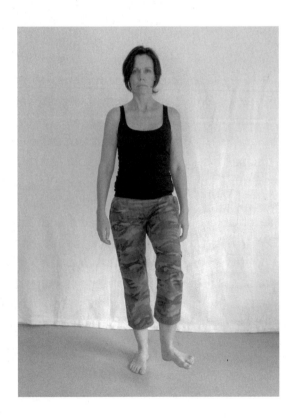

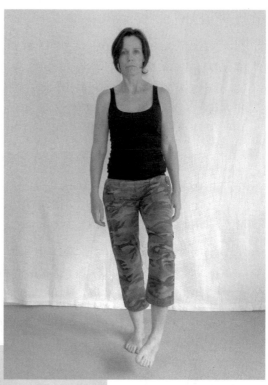

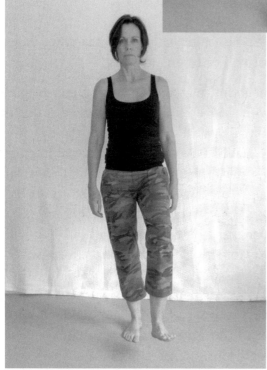

HANDS

The organ channels end or start at the fingers, so it is crucial to keep these mobile. Stiff fingers will restrict Chi flow along the associated channel and the organ system will therefore be affected. Try some finger exercises for loosening finger joints and also some exercises for opening up the palm.

- Shake your hands as if they are a wet mop.

- After a while imagine you are throwing your fingers to the ground. If you do this with each finger in turn it will help free the channel associated with that finger.

- Move your hands slowly in a horizontal figure of eight at your pelvis. Take them in one direction for a while, then in the other.

- Stretch your palms by bringing them together, intertwining your fingers and pushing the palms out from the centre of your chest.

- Hold each finger in turn and gently rotate it with the other hand, try to loosen all three finger joints.

In Chi Kung movement forms, beginners are often encouraged to follow their hands with their eyes and their awareness. If you think about it, this is actually what we do most of the day. We relate our minds to our hands in work tasks and social interactions. Reading, writing, typing, making things, doing things, all increase this relationship. Your awareness is mostly caught up with your hands and so, when you start practising Chi Kung, Chi flow will mostly be experienced in the hands and head. You will notice that you get most Chi effects in the centre of your hands. Perhaps they get hot, tingly, sweaty or prickly.

Expanding your awareness is imperative, as you need to have an equal connection with your whole body and mind, and not just one part of it. This will take time to build, but the first step is to make sure the hands are loose. Tension in the hands will trap

Chi and make it difficult for Chi to flow along the channels in the arms. The fingers are key structures, because of the channels that start or finish here. There are many exercises for loosening finger joints in Chi Kung. Try not to follow your hands in movements or over focus on them in static postures. Slowly your attention will disengage from them, and your mind will naturally expand and become interested in sensations and movements through the rest of the body. You will then realize how much of a tunnel vision you were holding in your hands.

ELBOWS AND KNEES

These joints are commonly ignored. In movement forms they are often stiff. It's best for the elbows to be soft, allowing the arms to have a flowing movement in forms. You might begin to notice that sometimes the elbows can lead a movement form or be pivotal in a static one. Here's an exercise to move Chi in the elbows.

Start the movement by bringing your hands up the centre line of the body and taking each hand in a circle out to the sides of the body and back down to the pelvis. As you make the movement, keep your elbows in a fixed position and let the forearms do most of the moving. The movement feels as if your forearms are the hands of a clock. After a while, change directions so the hands are coming down the centre line.

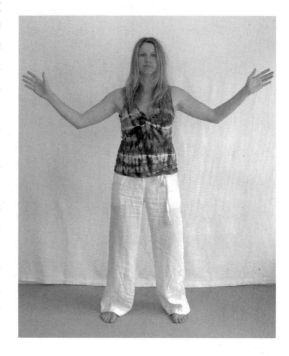

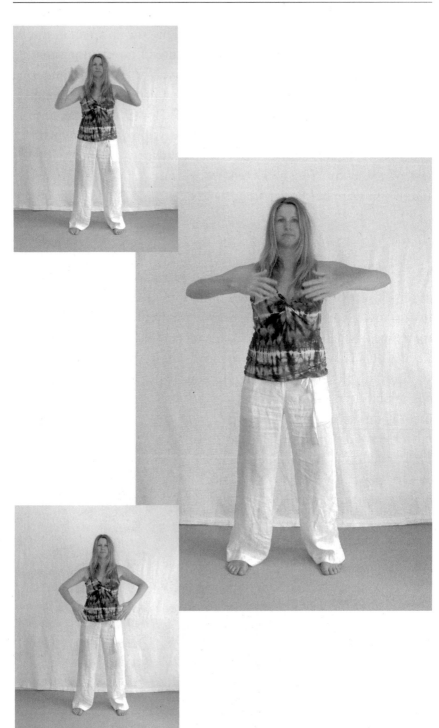

Most people suffer from painful knees because of all the strain in them from poor posture or from past injuries. You are encouraged in Chi Kung to move with lots of reference to the knees, to move carefully, and always move with the knees flexed. Locking the knees stops Chi flow and prevents fluid movement. Next time you walk down the street, be aware of your knees and how well they are bending. As you become more proficient in Chi Kung you will have less pain in your joints.

Bring your hands onto your knees. Loosely grip the knees with your fingers and lean into the knees with some of your upper body weight. Then take your knees in a circular pathway with both knees moving in the same direction. Make sure your feet and knees are touching so it feels as if you have one leg. As you circle the knees you will need to flex around each knee joint to allow the movement to take place. After a minute of this, take the movement in the opposite direction.

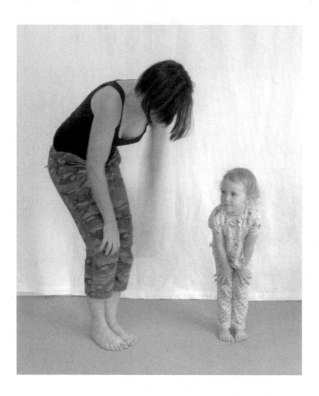

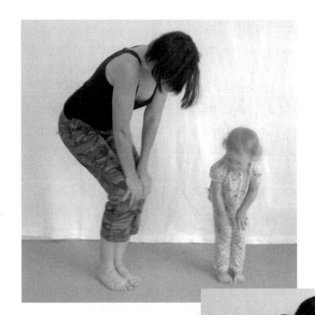

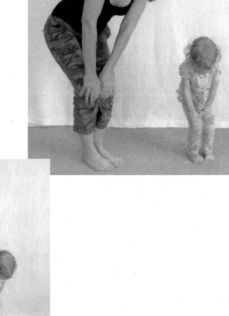

SHOULDERS AND HIPS

If the shoulder joints are restricted in any way, the whole arm will be compromised. The shoulders are the master joints for the arms, so lots of time should be spent exercising and loosening them up to allow Chi to flow across them more easily. The shoulders affect the hips. The hips are the master joints for the legs, and lots of emphasis should be given to loosening them up too. Like the shoulders, they can become tight and lose their freedom of movement. Circling movements are the most common exercise for both these joints.

For the shoulders, take the arms in big circles front to back that create a stretch into the muscles and tendons of the joint. Alternate the arms, so that you shift your weight from one leg to another and involve the Dan Tien. Make sure your wrists and elbows are soft in the movement. Try to make full circles even if you have to turn your chest.

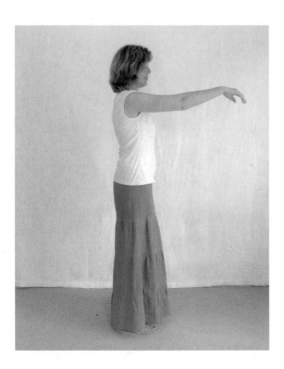

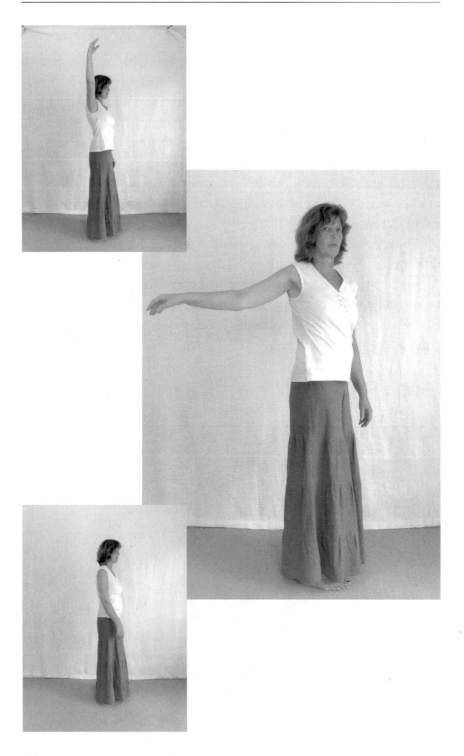

For the hips, balance on one leg and let your hands hang down by the sides of your pelvis. Take the leg in a circular movement so that the leg rises to right angles with the body and then moves out to the side. Let the lower leg hang, so that you take the knee up, out and down.

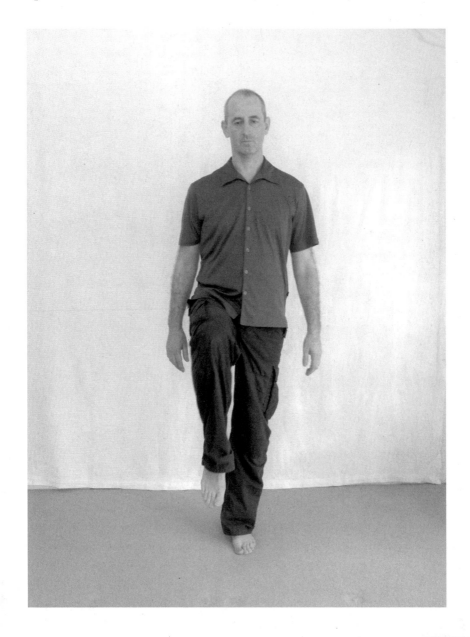

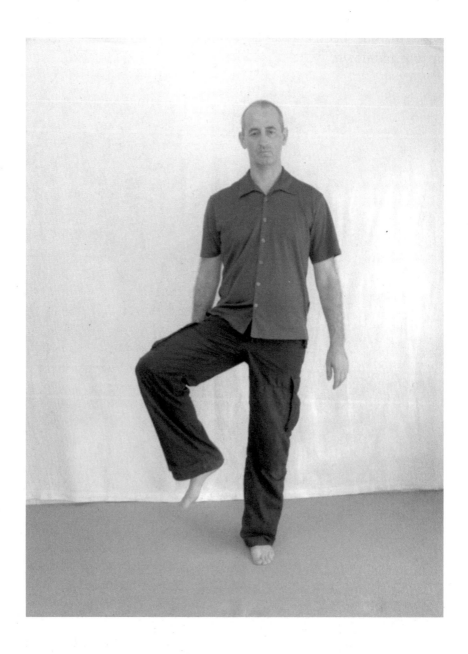

Chapter 10

CHI
FLOW

If you, in reaching this chapter, have been practising the forms described in the previous chapters, then you are ready to do the real thing. There are many approaches to Chi Kung and many different movement forms, ranging from the simple to the complex. However, they all have a set of fundamental movement principles.

OPENING MOVEMENT

Essentially this is a movement where the hands rotate outwards to show the palms, opening out in front of a particular structure. This movement can be used for an organ, the Dan Tien or any place in the body. It's the same movement.

For the heart, an opening movement comes about by placing the hands in front of the centre of the chest, palms looking towards the chest, then slowly rotating the hands and widening them out so they face away from the body. The intention is to relate the heart to the space in front of us and to the field in front of the body. Typically, there is then a flux between the field and the heart, which after some time tries to balance out. Initially there is a flurry of Chi movements that either settles down as things become balanced or, if there is a restriction that prevents this, Chi either can't move or circles around a particular area. Practising this form will reveal how your system is and provide an opportunity for the body tissues to adjust, and for Chi to move more freely. Much of Chi Kung is about discovering how your body/Chi system is, so that you can then begin to have a perspective of how Chi wants to move and express itself.

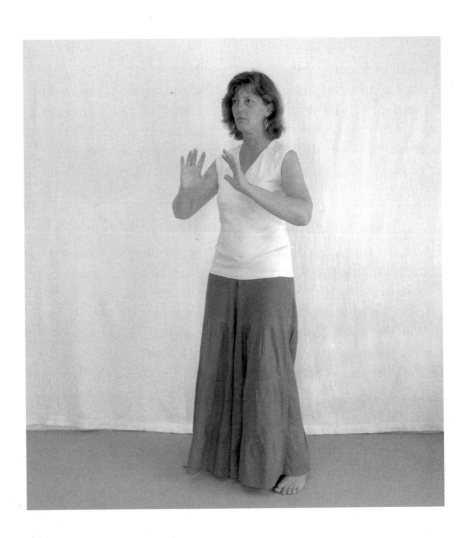

GATHERING MOVEMENTS

These movements act as the opposite of the opening forms. The emphasis here is on setting up a flow of external Chi moving into a place inside the body, for example the Dan Tien.

A classic form is to take the hands out from the pelvis and angle them so that the palms look at the centre of the pelvis. When you make the link with the Dan Tien, there is an automatic movement of Chi towards it, and a sense of Chi gathering into the core of the pelvis. This creates a more internal relationship with Chi whereby it circulates within the body.

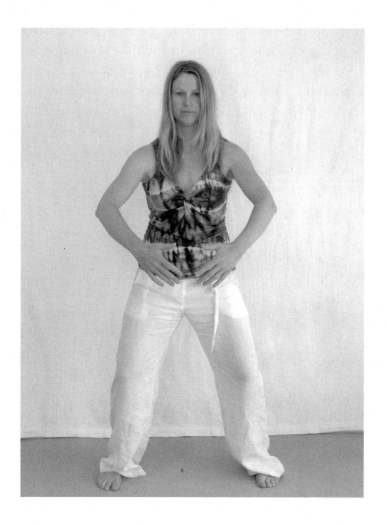

BALANCING LEFT AND RIGHT

Balancing the two sides of the body is an important aspect of Chi Kung. We often carry patterns of compression or strain in one side of the body that create difficulties in posture and movement, along with a reduced flow of Chi. Teaching the body to move out of these patterns is a vital part of Chi Kung. A common form is the movement of hands, moving, like lifts, in opposite directions. This movement not only simulates the natural Chi flows that move up and down the body, but also brings right and left sides of the body into harmony.

Start with the hands around the centre of the torso at the solar plexus, and face one palm up and one palm down. Now move them in the opposite direction to each other, along the length of the body, offset from each other by a couple of hand-widths. The hand that rises needs to twist and move faster to reach the full extension of the arm above the head. For a second, one hand

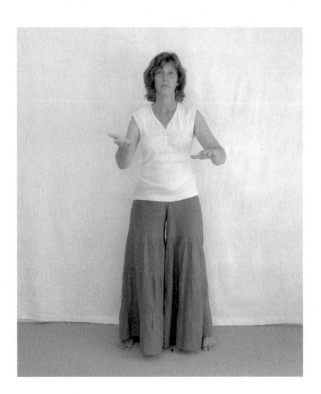

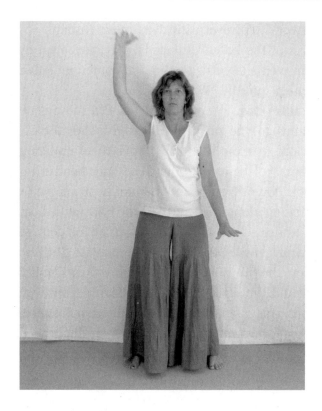

is at the pelvis and the other above the head and the palms are looking to the sky and the earth. Flip the hands at the wrists and move each in the opposite direction, allowing the hands to pass each other at the solar plexus at the same time. Continuing with this exercise will equalize Chi flow on your left and right sides.

BALANCING UP AND DOWN

Balancing out the flow of Chi along the length of the body is one of the main intentions of Chi Kung. For greater health and strength there must be free, unimpeded flow along the length of the body from the feet to the head. The body should also have the ability to allow Chi to flow from head to toe. Much of this movement takes place in the body's connective tissue framework, in the same way that blood and nervous impulses flow through this network. However, Chi does move through all tissues and structures of the body. Ultimately, this movement up and down allows heaven and earth to join and come into balance, creating a deepening into the "Wu Chi" state.

A simple form to encourage this Chi movement is to bring your hands to the pelvis, with your palms looking up (keep hands close to the centre line), move them up along the length of the body to the top of your head and then turn them so that they look down. Now move the hands down the length of the body, sinking along the length of the body at the same time, and repeat. Notice which movement is easier for you – up or down – and which movement creates the greater Chi response. After practising this for some time the movements will balance out. Note we did the same exercise in Chapter 1 but with a different intention. This is an example of using your Yi (mind intention), so that the form looks physically the same but because of your Yi the stimulation of Chi within it is quite different.

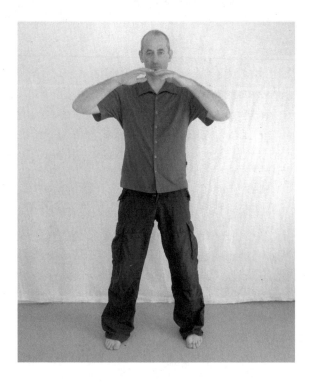

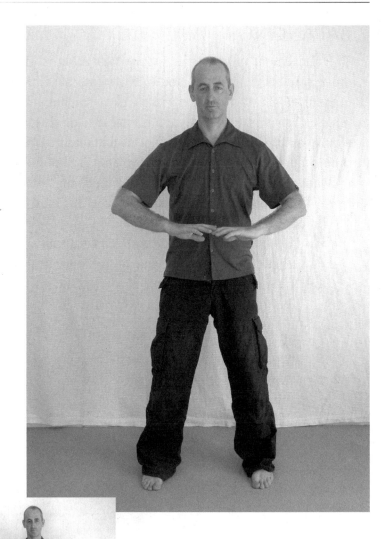

BALANCING IN AND OUT

This movement of Chi is necessary for taking in Chi from the universal field around you, and to allow internal Chi to dissipate. Sometimes Chi can build up in parts of the body and needs to release outwards. If your system is unable to do this, there will be a build up of Chi in the body and resultant aggravation. An ideal state occurs when there is free movement, not only between the universal field and yours, but also between your internal and external fields. This movement will promote this ideal relationship.

Simply bring the hands to anywhere along the centre line of the torso and, with palms leading, push them outwards into the space in front of you and sink your body, bending the knees and keeping the back straight. Keep the hands at the same level of the body. Then bring the hands in slowly, palms leading.

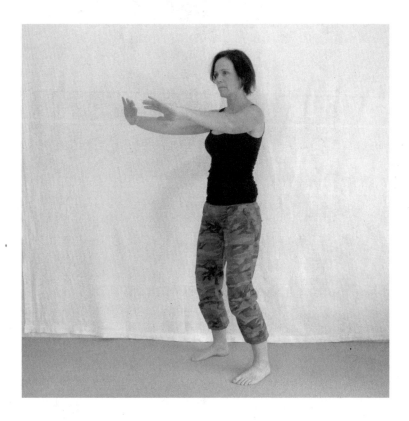

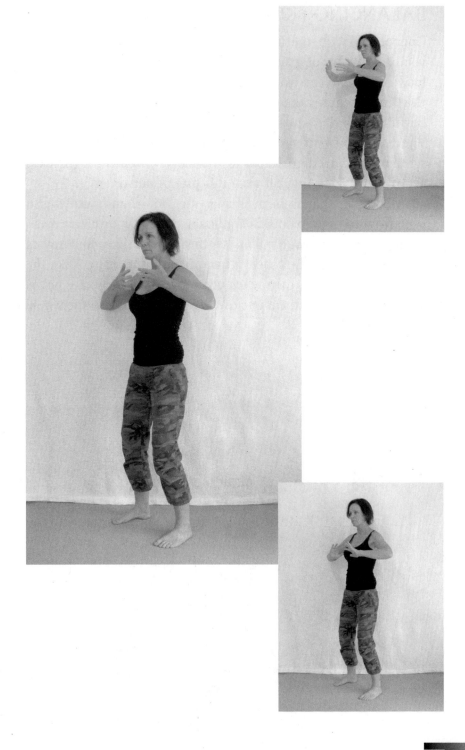

BALANCING FRONT AND BACK

Connecting with the back of the body and the space behind you can be a bit of a surprise. Most of our awareness is focused forwards and to the front of the body, so the back gets ignored. Chi Kung believes there is a large Chi field behind us that can be utilized, and is a powerful space where lots of our energy lies. The more you become aware of this, the more you open your system to connecting deeply to this field. Often through stress and trauma we can cut off from this part of ourselves.

Move your hands in a circular motion around your waist, from front to back, palms facing down; then as your hands reach behind you, turn your palms, so that it feels like your hands are scooping from the space out and behind the waist. Take the hands out wide first, then when you move them forwards, palms looking front, bring them in close to the waist. Sink in the whole body as you do this.

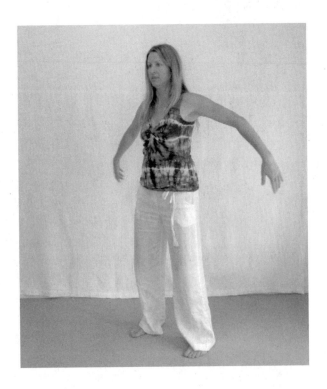

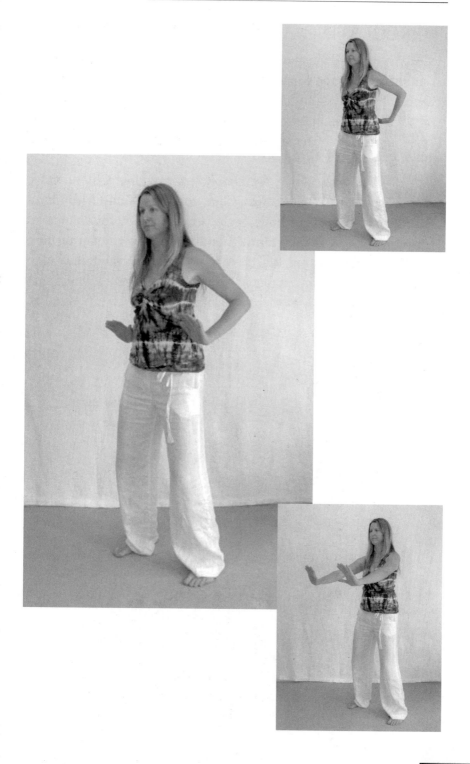

CIRCULATING ALONG THE BODY

Flow is often in loops or circuits, and stimulating Chi to move in circuits is a classic concept. There are a number of circuits in the body that allow Chi to flow along the body. There are circuits that connect the limbs, circuits that connect the axis of the body, plus an urge for Chi to flow freely along the full length of the body in a circuit.

Here's a great form for simply encouraging Chi to move throughout the whole system. Take your hands into a windmill movement across your body in one direction. Let your hands go as high and low as they can without bending down or stretching up. Don't move too quickly. Slow movements that you follow with your mind's attention engage Chi flow best. Imagine a wheel, and imagine that your arms are spokes of the wheel. You can visualize

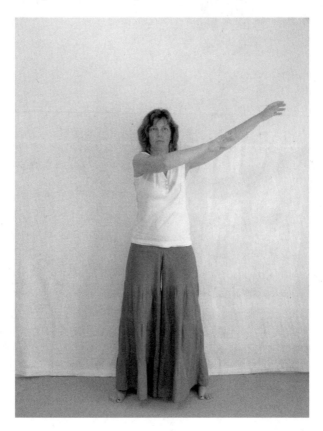

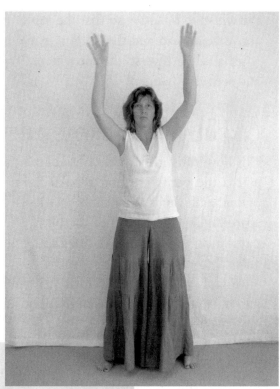

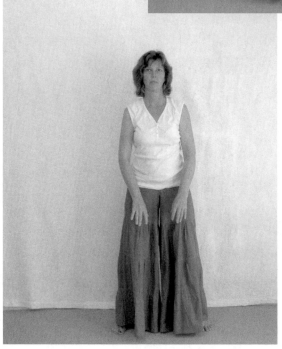

the wheel to be large, so that the top of it is moving in the space above your head and the bottom is moving through the ground. After a while reverse the movement. Try this form very slowly and see what happens.

CIRCULATING ACROSS THE BODY

Chi flow runs in currents horizontally along circular pathways across the body, creating a balance in the horizontal plane. A pivotal pathway is at the umbilicus level, but there are many more spaced along the length of the body. Working with the circular pathway at the umbilicus brings about movement in all the pathways above and below this level.

Simply make a circular form in front of your body with your hands, palms down in front of the abdomen. Imagine the pathway

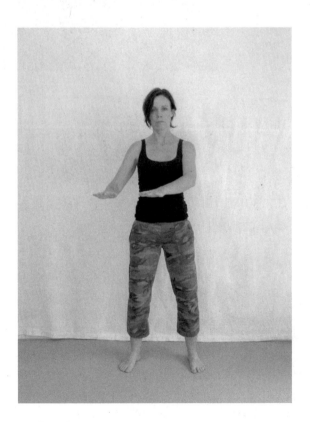

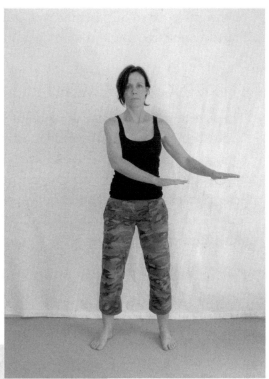

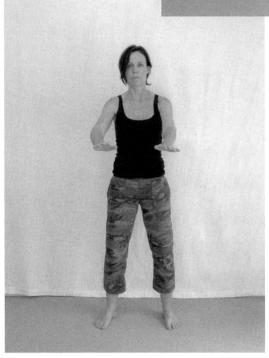

YOU ARE HOW YOU MOVE

of the circle extending behind you like an equator of the body. Start in one direction and then try it in the opposite direction.

FLOWING MOVEMENT

Think of water and allow the quality of the water to enter your body. The body is highly fluid, so this should create a strong connection. As you practise Chi Kung forms, let your body take on this quality, so that your movement is informed by the characteristics of flow, ease and smoothness. In time your movements will become seamless and you will glide through forms in the way water flows in a river.

Chapter 11

FIRE
AND WATER

A few thousand years ago in China, sages, philosophers and practitioners of introspection looked for explanations of the world they experienced around and within themselves. They came up with a theory of the existence of elements hidden behind the external fabric of nature. This theory has come in different forms and sizes over the centuries, but has now gathered into a generally accepted paradigm called "the theory of the five elements or five transformations". In a nutshell, it says that behind all things there are five elements, (Fire, Water, Earth, Metal and Wood) according to which you can classify all things in nature. Most Chi Kung practices are based on this theory. The elements are often organized into the following relationships, which show how they interact and transform from one element into another and how they create balance between each other.

The idea is that none of these elements are fixed, they are all in a state of flux, just like the universe. Everything changes constantly from one state into another.

The elements most commonly associated in Chi Kung are Fire and Water. These elements in many ways represent the balance of yin and yang in the body and they are often worked with together to create harmony. If there is harmony in the Fire–Water elements, then the other elements will follow suit. The important

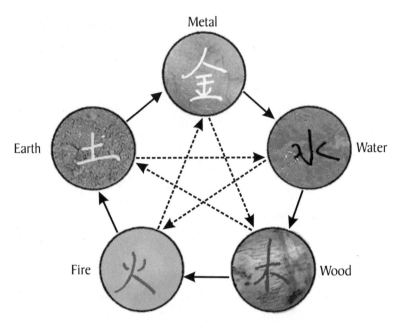

The five elements

thing for the Chi Kung practitioner is the elemental relationships within the body. You only have control over these forces. Once you are able to achieve a balanced state, you will begin to affect the world and the people around you in movement towards an equally balanced state.

FIRE AND WATER IN THE BODY

The action of Fire and Water in the body is both opposite and complementary. There are a lot of complex definitions of the elements available in Traditional Chinese Medicine, but the Chi Kung practitioner seeks simplicity. The simple approach is Water cools – Fire warms. Water likes to descend and Fire likes to rise, so the lower body is more associated with Water and the upper with Fire. We need both, otherwise our systems will be out of balance. The most common imbalance is too much Fire. This is not a great position to be in, as it creates an experience of everything moving too fast, overheating, emotional overwhelm and lack of groundedness. Look around you and you will notice many people exhibiting these conditions. It's a very common trend in the modern world. The solution is to spend time making a strong relationship to Water in your body. This is the major focus of most Chi Kung approaches. When Water is expressing itself in your Chi system, then Fire will automatically become harmonious. Find out how these elements are in you. Here is a simple diagnosis that comes in two parts.

Standing, place your hands at the level of your diaphragm and turn your hands so that your palms look upwards towards Fire. Stay like this for a minute and notice if there are any responses from your body – such as any sensations, or movements in body structures, Chi movements, or changes in your mind state. Now turn your palms so that they look down towards Water. Same thing again, notice any responses. Which one responded the most?

Now do a movement form. Bring your hands as low as they will go in front of the thighs. Imagine your hands are scooping under the soles of your feet, by making a scooping action, and take your hands up to the level of your waist, leading with your palms, then turn them and go back the way you came in front of the pelvis and legs. Repeat a few times and notice any response. Do a similar movement in the upper body. Bring your hands to the centre of your chest and let the palms face each other. Slowly draw the hands apart and let them rise, so your hands end up out to the sides of your head, with the palms looking upwards. Reverse the movement and repeat.

Now you should be able to make a diagnosis of your Fire–Water balance. Don't be surprised if it is Fire that responded more, and Water less. If the responses for each were similar then please feel free to go around telling your friends and family about it, as there's probably no need for you to attend a Chi Kung class!

WATER ELEMENT FORMS, ORGAN FORMS, ANIMAL FORMS

There are many forms that fit into these categories, but here are three that exemplify the quality and movement of Water and, if practised, will lead to a strengthening of this element within you.

Sea form

Using the image of the sea will help you connect with Water Chi. Standing with one foot forward, draw your hands from your pelvis so that they move forward as you shift your weight to the front leg, bring the hands up to waist height, face the palms forward, and push the hands gently but firmly into the space in front of you, keeping them low. As you shift your weight back,

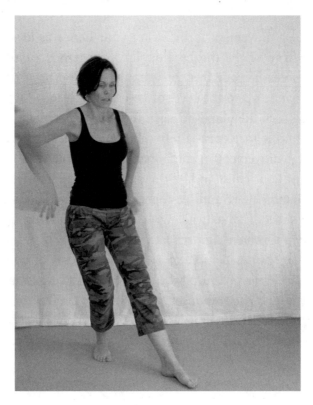

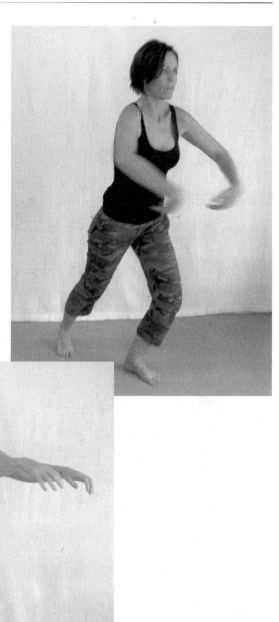

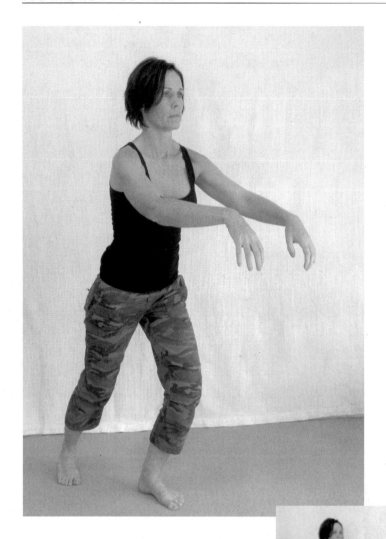

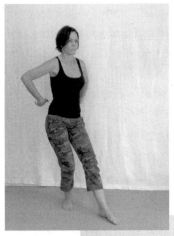

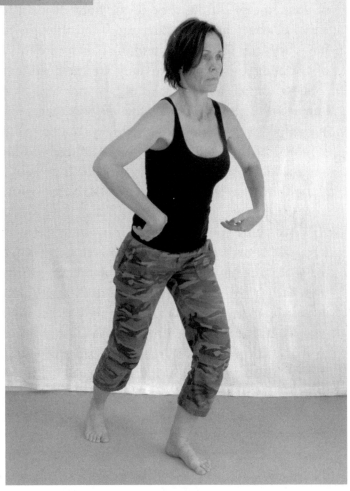

flex the wrists and draw the hands in to the body by the sides of the pelvis and behind you. The movement is meant to mimic the ebb and flow of the sea. Imagine that you are casting a fishing net out in front of you when you push forward, and drawing the net back towards you when you shift your weight back. Try the form with your other foot forward.

Kidney form

A good way to feel your kidney Chi is to bring your hands and place them on your kidneys. Your kidneys are at the bottom of your ribcage, at the back of the body at waist level. Put the backs of your hands on them and listen through your hands to how they feel. The kidneys and the bladder are the Water organs of the body. Organs in Chi Kung are classified into "solid" and "hollow" organs and the solid organs are considered to be more important. The solid organs are the yin organs and when yin is changed, yang follows. The kidneys are the solid, yin organ, so many of the Water forms orient around the kidney organs and the kidney channel, which runs from the bottom of the feet, along the inside of the legs, and up the torso – just out from the front centre line.

Check how your kidney Chi is by doing a kidney form. This form will stimulate your kidney Chi. Bring your hands out into the space directly in front of your umbilicus, palms facing away from each other, and take them out to the sides and behind you, in a circle. It feels as if you are swimming or parting curtains. Put your hands behind the kidneys and let the hands and wrists turn so that you bring your hands to the sides of your waist, palms forward. Now push forwards through the waist, and sink your body, flexing the knees and keeping the body upright. Move the hands forward, and make sure they stay at kidney height. As you reach the furthest point away from the body in front of you, move the hands out to the sides in a circular pathway back to the kidneys and, as you do this, your body slightly rises as you

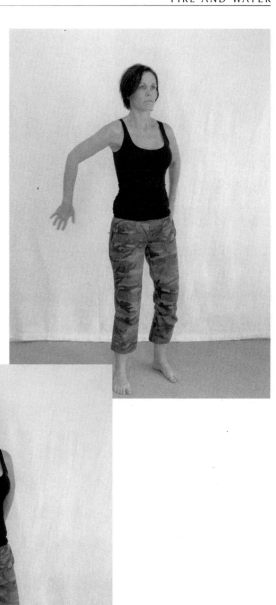

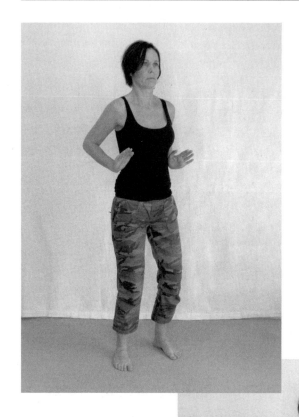

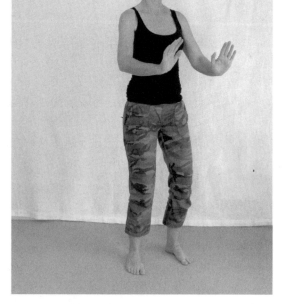

breathe in. This should feel as if you are gathering Chi into the kidneys. Bring the hands, through the waist, palms front, and sink again, but this time synchronize your out-breath with the movement. Breathe in as your hands go back. The whole circular form is one breath cycle. Keep repeating the movement until you feel a movement of Chi in the body. It shouldn't take long, as the form is strong and can quickly gather and move your Chi. You might notice this form is very similar to the balancing front and back form in Chapter 10. Using similar forms for different effects is a common event in Chi Kung.

Bear form

If you've ever been to a zoo or watched documentaries of bears you will see why this animal was chosen to represent the Water element. The Bear is powerful, and its centre of gravity is low and close to the ground. Water has a downward energy and seeks to flow to the lowest point. Water is irresistible in its pathway.

Find a place to stand quietly, and bring both hands to the centre of your torso. Turn your hands into loose fists and spread your legs into a wide stance and sink. Make sure your arms are rounded, with elbows sticking out to the sides. Now imagine that you are a Bear. Contemplate the qualities and appearance of a Bear, and as you do this your body and Chi will start to take on the shape and energy of the Bear. The more you do this, the stronger the connection becomes. This is a Bear standing posture that will generate a lot of Chi in the pelvis and lower body.

You can progress this form into a Bear walk by keeping your hands static and shifting your weight from one leg to another like a Sumo wrestler. Keep a wide stance and, when you step, bring all your body weight into the step and at the last second slap the floor with your foot. This will sink your Chi and wake up "bubbling spring" at the centre of the sole of the foot. Walk like this for a few minutes and then come back to the stationary posture. Visualize the Bear again, and notice what has changed.

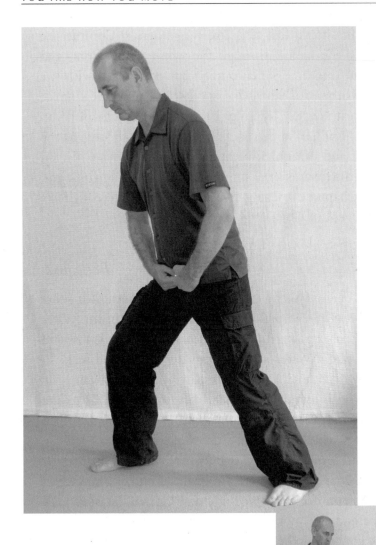

FIRE ELEMENT FORMS, ORGAN FORMS, ANIMAL FORMS

There are possibly even more Fire than Water forms, but here are three that are representative and will help you access your Fire Chi.

Flame Form

A simple way to experience Fire is to envisage flames in your body. It's amazing how strongly your body takes this up. Stand with your hands crossed in front of your heart. Imagine flames flickering up your legs and through your torso up to your chest. After a

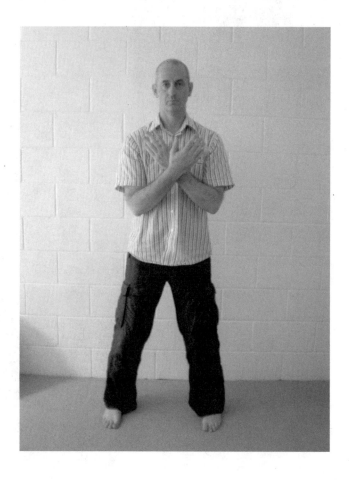

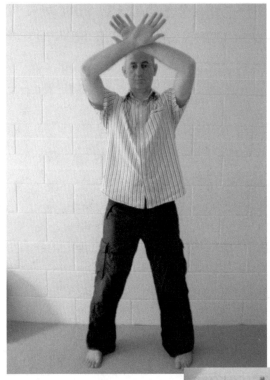

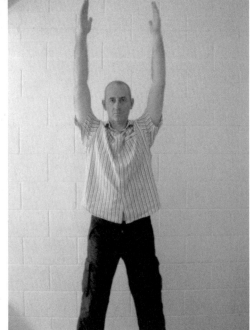

minute of this, move your hands up in front of your forehead and let your hands rotate so your palms look forward. Imagine the flames licking up through your neck and into your head. After a minute of this, take your hands above your head and straighten your arms so they are perpendicular, fingers looking up to the sky. Now imagine the flames licking up the length of your arms. Stay with it for another minute and then take your hands down and let go of the image. Now stand and feel the Fire Chi in you.

Heart form

The heart is the chief Fire organ. Its channels run from the centre of the armpits along the inside of the arms to the small fingers. Internally there are connections directly to the heart. A heart form balances Fire in the upper body and brings about a rhythm, not just in the heart itself, but throughout the whole system. Blood is a strong Chi in the body and its successful circulation depends on the strength and internal balance of the heart organ. The following exercise both stimulates the heart channels to create a smooth flow and regulates the heart so that its beat becomes less erratic and more orderly.

Bring your hands into a cupped prayer position in front of your heart; stay in this posture for a while until the Chi thickens and streams between your hands. Then roll the hands forward so that the fingertips face forwards, and widen the hands out from each other so that the palms keep looking at each other, across the chest, until the arms are at maximum stretch. Then turn the wrists so that the palms look forward. This movement should feel like an expansion of the chest. Now the elbows drop and the hands come back together, palms looking at each other again, but the hands are now vertical – fingertips looking up to the sky. Bring the hands back into the centre of the chest where they began. On the next repetition, combine the movement with your breath, breathing in as you expand the space between your palms. That should feel like the natural thing to do. As you drop

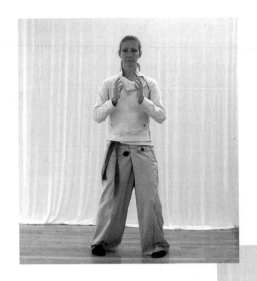

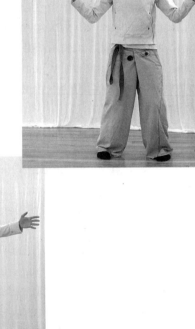

your elbows, start to breathe out. On the next repetition, sink as you breathe out and rise as you breathe in. Your whole body should feel as if it is involved in the movement, not just the hands and arms. Stay with the form for five minutes, then stand still, with your hands facing each other at the centre of your chest. How does the Chi feel now?

Crane form

The Fire animal is the Bird. An indigenous Chinese bird is the crane, which has a large wing-span and long legs and is very graceful. Just like the Bear, the idea here is to allow yourself, through the image, to resonate with the qualities of the Crane. Fire rises, spreads and disperses and the crane should feel light and able to rise. When you do Crane forms you should imagine your arms are wings. Start in a Crane pose by bringing all your fingertips together with the tip of your thumb, and taking your hands out to the sides of your head, like wings. Let the wrists be softly flexed, and be strong between the shoulder blades and spine. Stay in the stance for a couple of minutes, using the image of the Crane, with your arms being like wings, then shift into a movement form. Let your hands descend in an oblique angle, towards the centre of your pelvis, and as you do this, slowly open your hands until your fingers are spread and the centre of your palms are showing; let your wrists flex in the opposite direction. When your hands reach the centre of the pelvis, start to synchro-nize your breath with the arm movements. So, breathe in as your hands and arms ascend back up to the Crane pose, letting the back of your wrists lead and gathering your fingertips together until you come back to the original position. Breathe out as your wings descend, slightly sinking. You can progress this movement into a walk: simply shift your weight to one leg on the in-breath as your wings rise, and step as your wings descend. Stay with your natural breath, do the walk in time to this. As you master the walk you can feel very light and spacious, with a wonderful

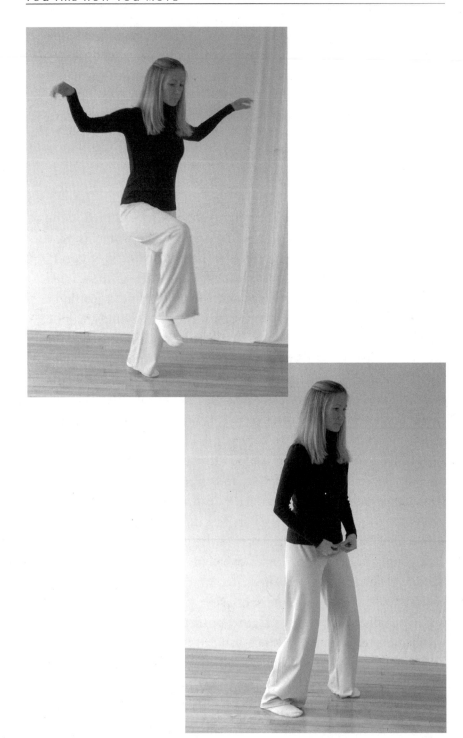

flow of Chi moving through and around you. When you have walked for a few minutes come back to the original standing Crane pose. Rest in this pose for a couple of minutes and notice how your body is and where the Chi flows.

WORKING WITH FIRE AND WATER

This is the heart of Chi Kung. Use these forms to create stronger expressions of these energies in your body. Try alternating the forms, so move from kidney to heart forms. Start with one, then shift to another and see if you can bring them into a fuller relationship with each other. At first you will notice one is predominant, but as time and practice go on, they should both become fuller and more balanced. Try walking like a Bear, then like a Crane, then back to the Bear. Transitioning like this gets your system used to the two elements combining. This in turn affects the make-up and balance of your whole system. Water governs the nervous system, bones and Jing (your constitutional energy); Fire governs blood and Shen (your spiritual energy).

Chapter 12

TRANSFORMATIONS

The aim of Chi Kung is to ignite the central channels of energy so that Chi is flowing around a central orbit and up a central channel. The Taoist mystical theory that underlies Chi Kung practice is consistent with many other mystical traditions in holding that within the body there is a central channel that has a rising energy and two other energy channels that balance the central one. In Chi Kung the central channel is called Chong Mai, and the two balancing channels form a front and back orbit around the torso and head, around Chong Mai. The ultimate goal in Chi Kung is to create flow in the orbit. When this becomes established the central channel, Chong Mai, activates and Chi starts to flow more strongly through it, and you form a deeper connection to the Tao. Organized along the Chong Mai are a number of Dan Tiens that are centres of Chi. The three main Dan Tiens are approximately positioned in the head, the heart area, and the lower belly. (So far you have been connecting with the lowest Dan Tien at the pelvis in previous exercises.) This is a primary energy system at the core of the body and is surrounded by the organ system. Chi Kung work involves strengthening and loosening the body to create Chi flow. The organs of the body are worked with specifically, to remove excess Chi, or stagnant or deficient Chi, so that each arrives at a balanced state. There are many forms, but most of them follow the organ channel systems. As the organ energies start to become healthier, the central channels start to enliven. Doing central channel exercises encourages a stronger Chi movement in the core of the body. As the Chi movement strengthens, the front and back orbit start to flow, activating Chong Mai and deepening the connection to the Tao. This happens gradually and can be experienced as a progressive feeling of centredness, energy, and creativity. As this channel starts to flow more powerfully, and your connection to the Tao deepens, your life begins to become informed by the Tao and your consciousness moves in line with it. The Chi Kung practitioner can work directly with the central orbits which are together called the microcosmic orbit, to encourage this transformation in consciousness. The organ systems also need to be worked with, so that there is a holistic shift in your Chi state.

When you examine the origins of early life and how we form ourselves embryologically, you can observe that the first structures to appear are fluid-filled spaces, at the centre of which lies the precursor of our spine and central nervous system. Once this is established, the organs start to appear. This is consistent with the paradigm in Chi Kung that the central channels are deeper and more primary than the organ systems. The central channels are composed of an inner core of eight channels, called the "eight extraordinary vessels". The first to form in the embryo is the centre-most vessel, called "Chong Mai" or the "thrusting channel". The movement associated with this channel is a rising current, moving from the bottom of the spine at the coccyx to the top of the head. The two channels organized as an orbital circuit around it are the "Ren" and "Du" channels, often known as the "Conception" and "Governing" vessels. Chi circulates in this orbit, most commonly in a direction that is up the back and down the front. The Governing vessel is mostly associated with the nervous system, and the Conception with the organs. These three channels are the innermost channels and are not connected to the channels of the organ system; they remain independent of them and act like a reservoir or "sea of Chi", either absorbing excess Chi from the organ system or providing Chi when there

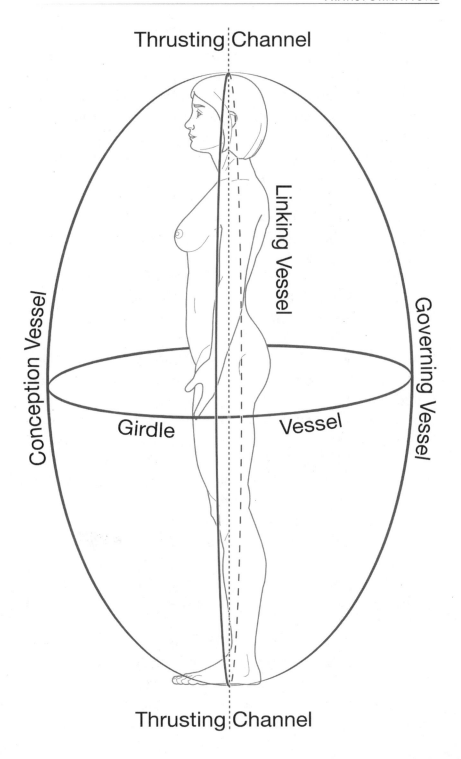

Thrusting Channel

Linking Vessel

Conception Vessel

Governing Vessel

Girdle Vessel

Thrusting Channel

is depletion. So the Chi in these channels represents a core Chi. Often these channels lie dormant, but can, through Chi Kung practice, become empowered and bring the whole system to a much higher state of energy, vitality and consciousness. The three Dan Tiens are particularly associated with these core channels and as your practice matures the Dan Tiens emanate more powerfully in the body and in the body's energy field, creating elevated states of mind and perception.

Out from the innermost channels, there is the Girdle or Belt channel, which is arranged around the waist, horizontally crossing the umbilicus at the front. This channel helps balance the horizontal Chi flows in the body in the same way as the first three balance the vertical flows. The channel has a strong relationship to the umbilicus.

The remaining channels are called the "linking vessels" and are oriented around the limbs, connecting the sides of the body with the lower limbs in particular, but also with the shoulders. They are like an orbit; each orbit being a composite of two linking vessels, just like the central microcosmic orbit which is a composite of the central vessels. However, these orbits are arranged at right angles to the microcosmic orbit; while the microcosmic orbit flows around the front and back of the body, these orbits flow around the sides of the body. When Chi flows in these orbits it helps to balance the sides of the body with the four limbs and also acts as a support for the microcosmic orbit. Together, these channels with the girdle provide a more direct link to the organ system.

You can practise a Chi Kung sequence that will help bring you into relationship to the movements of Chi in these central vessels.

Start from the outermost of these orbits (that is, the linking vessel orbits) and work your way into the centre-most channel.

Let your hand trace around the orbit from foot to shoulder, encouraging Chi to move up along the outer channel, then down the inner channel on the insides of the legs. Alternate the sides.

Linking vessel form

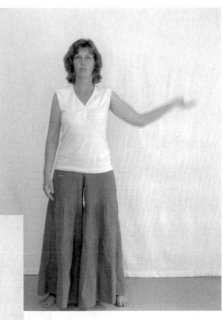

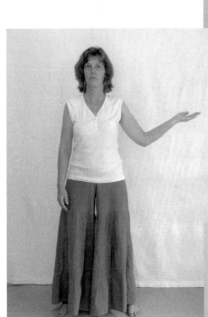

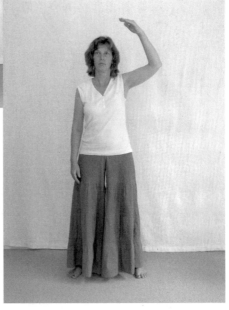

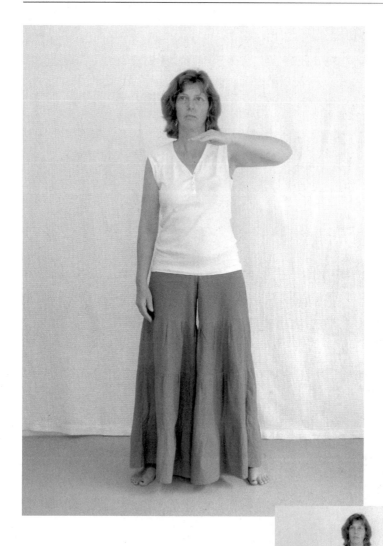

Stay with the movement for a while until you notice a smooth sense of flow on either side.

Then shift to the Girdle channel and make a horizontal circular movement in front and to the side of the body with your palms looking down. Imagine that the circle extends out from your waist in all directions around you and that your hands are moving along a track, like the equator of your body. Explore how far this field extends out from the body. As with the linking vessels, keep doing the movement until there's a sense of a smooth flow or at least a shift in the way Chi flows.

Then move to the microcosmic orbit. Start at the pelvis and take your hands, palms upwards, up the sides of the body, having an intention to connect with the back of your body and the channel along the spine. Your hands move up to the sides of your head, following the channel across the middle of your head, then follow the orbit down the front centre line all the way to the pelvis, and back up the sides again, again connecting with the channel rising up the spine. Make sure you don't do this too fast as the Chi field here is very sensitive. Try to sense at what pace and strength your movements should be. In time, as you practise, this orbit will start to flow more easily and you will become more aware of its field, until it's part of your daily experience.

Now shift your awareness to the central channel. Start with your hands at the pelvis, palms upwards, and let them slowly rise up through the length of the body's axis; let your hands rotate in front of your neck and face, and follow them above the head and back down the sides. Then repeat the form again. Stay with the form until there's a sense of a delicate rising force in you that makes you feel expansive. Your mind should naturally become still and you should spontaneously shift into a static standing posture. You can stop here or you can move back through the forms in reverse.

Orbit form

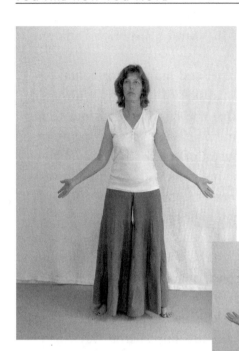

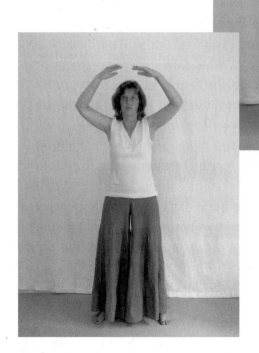

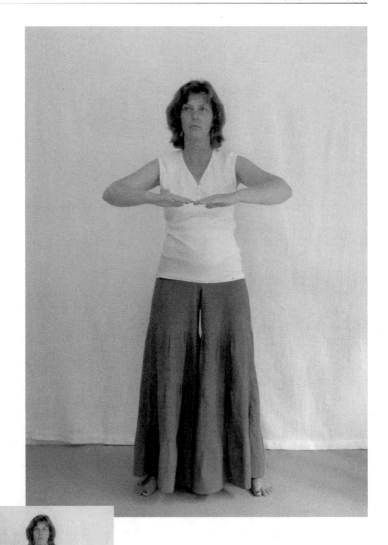

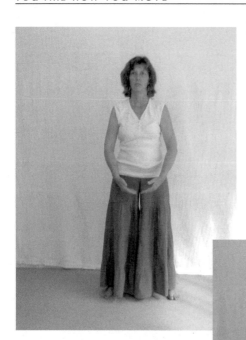

Chong Mai form

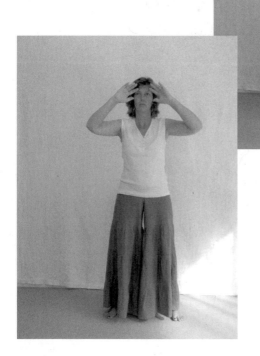

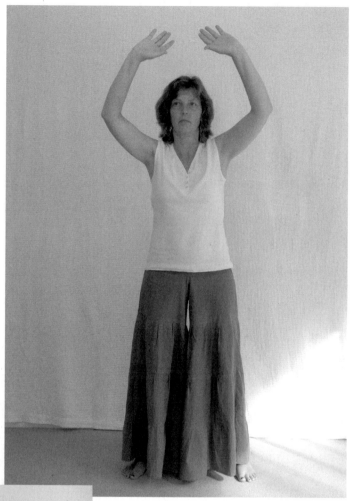

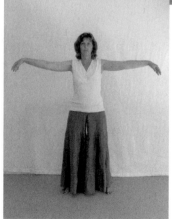

Chapter 13

BE SPONTANEOUS

Когда you become good at listening to your body and aware of the structures and spaces within and around you, you will be able to let your body express natural motion. This is the truly creative space of Chi Kung. The mature Chi Kung practitioner follows the Chi expressions in his practice, so that forms spontaneously emerge from a creative Chi space. Here are a few ways you can encourage this.

MOVING FROM STILLNESS

The purest form of spontaneous Chi Kung is to stand still and wait for the Chi to move you. The art of this consists in coming into an internal stillness and in being highly sensitive to Chi flow in and around you. You are getting in touch with an instinctual part of yourself. It's important to allow the whole body to be available to move, so that you can be spontaneous as a whole unit, not just a limb or a region being open to movement. Then you can express fully the flow of Chi. Doing this will make you creative. You are entering a creative space and fine tuning your skills of connecting to the subtle movements that are within you. Commonly, spontaneous adjustments take place in the body as you do this, which can make your body move in unusual ways.

VARYING FORMS

Take any of the movement forms in the book and rather than staying with the form, give your body permission to express it differently. It might be just a shift in nuance, so that you subtly alter a part of the form. It could be a different hand gesture or elevation of the arms. Keep letting go into how your body wants to move in the form. Let go of the structure of the form slowly, and allow more and more latitude for instinctual movement. In particular, listen to the Chi and where it wants to go, and let it move your body. As you deepen into the spontaneous state, the form may undergo a complete transformation into something else entirely. Or it may stay within its original boundaries and modify.

You can become skilled at letting go into the Chi and being sensitive to deeper movements within you. Forms spontaneously arise when you allow them to, and you drop into a world of unknowing. Each second, you are listening to how your body and Chi field want to express themselves, so you need to let go of expectations and rid yourself of predictable and habituated responses. This is not an easy thing to do. It's amazing how patterned we are as human beings and how we hold on to repetition and the known. So it can be challenging at first to allow these movements to come to the surface. When they do, you can feel emancipated, and you will be amazed by the kind of movements you will express. Often spiral and helical movements emerge, then sometimes you can feel like an animal and want to make sounds like one, or you can feel like a movement in nature, a river flowing, or the sea, or suddenly you might come to a stop and stand still like a mountain. Practising this approach is highly therapeutic and can be a fast road to connecting with the Tao. Letting go of your programming will rapidly change your view of yourself and the world around you. In this way, Chi Kung practice becomes revolutionary and transformational.

Chapter 14

CHI
MEDITATIONS

C hi Kung is full of remarkable meditations. These are in-
spired by the many different traditions linking Chi Kung
to Taoism, Buddhism, Traditional Chinese Medicine, shamanism,
Confucianism, nature, and all of the numerous schools of Chi
Kung and internal alchemy. Here is a list of some of the more
remarkable ones.

THE LAKE

Imagine you are sitting on the banks of a lake. Be open to whatever image comes to you. Visualize the lake being choppy on the
surface as the wind is blowing clouds across it. As the wind begins
to drop in its intensity you notice the surface starts to settle. As
the wind drops even more you begin to see below the surface
of the lake. Silt begins to drop towards the bottom and strong
currents and eddies start to slow down. Suddenly, the wind stops
and the clouds depart and the surface becomes smooth. Under
the surface you can see into the depths of the lake. The whole
body of water can be seen and felt as still and tranquil. Notice the
effects this visualization has on your body and mind.

WATERFALL

Find a quiet place to stand. Imagine you are standing underneath a waterfall. Let the water flow down the back of your head, along the back of your body, the back of your legs, and over the front of your feet, before flowing into the ground. The water is following the course of the bladder channel, which runs down through the central plane of the head and, like tramlines, down the back – one tramline either side of the spine. Let the water be cool and refreshing. As you stay with the images, open up to the Chi effect. Where do you feel Chi movements? How does your body respond? The most common effect is to feel revitalized and grounded.

THE RIVER

Find a quiet place to stand. Imagine you are standing in a river. Visualize the water being up to your waist. You are facing the direction of the flow and in order to stand firmly in the current you need to sink and become heavy in your feet. Lean forward a little, so you are leaning into the current. Feel the flow of water coursing over your legs and pelvis. Stay like this for a while and then turn around so that you are facing away from the flow of water, and lean back a little into the current. This is a meditation for bringing Chi into the lower body and for sinking your Chi downwards.

FIRE AND WATER

Find a quiet place to sit. It's important you sit in whatever position you feel comfortable. It could be sitting on a chair, or a cushion or a stool, or in cross legs. Make sure your spine is erect and you can let your body relax. Come into whole body awareness. Once this is established, bring your awareness into your pelvis until you can feel sensation in the area. Imagine that the pelvis is half-filled with clear, cool water. Just like the lake meditation, this is your internal lake. Notice how it is. See if you can bring it into a state of still waters by calming your body and mind, and envisioning the waters as still. Stay with it for a while and then let the image dissolve and replace it with an image of a flame, at the very centre of your pelvis. Sit watching the flame for a while, and notice the effect it has on your mind and body, and how different it is to water. Now imagine the water returns and the flame transforms into a floating candle flame. The flame remains at the centre of the lake. Notice how bringing them together creates a whole new dynamic. This is a great meditation for focusing the mind and creating balance in fire and water, plus, of course, for stimulating the lower Dan Tien.

TREE

Find a quiet place to stand, if possible next to some trees. Start with your legs wide (at least two hip-widths apart) and put your hands out in front of your pelvis, palms facing towards your body. Imagine your legs and arms wrapping around the trunk of a tree. Let the strength of the tree support you in the standing posture. Use the tree to connect downwards into the earth through the roots. Stay like this for a couple of minutes, then bring your arms higher up to the level of your chest and reconnect to the image. This time not only form a relationship downwards using the image of the root system, but also upwards into the canopy of the tree, visualizing the branches and leaves in your mind's eye. Notice the Chi quality and flow.

MUD STATUE

Find a quiet place to stand, preferably outside on the ground. Imagine that your body is made of mud. Give your body time to respond to the image. It should give you a feeling of heaviness and connection to the ground. The visualization is trying to open you up to the Chi of the earth element. Now bring one of your hands up to the level of your head and one down to your pelvis, both palms look forward. Imagine that the mud starts to dry out, so that you become like a clay statue. This should make you feel very still and unmoving. If your upper arm becomes tired, switch hands so that the other hand becomes the higher one.

TAI CHI

Find a quiet place to sit. Sit comfortably. Close your eyes and make a conscious connection to your body sensations throughout the whole of your body. Stay with that for a couple of minutes, then open your eyes and acknowledge the space around you. Half close your eyes and be with a sense of both. This will bring you into a relationship with your internal and external Chi. Imagine at the centre of your pelvis there is a Tai Chi disc. Let it start as a small circle at the centre of your pelvis. Watch the way the yin and yang, the black and white embryonic shapes, curl around each other. After a while, imagine that the disc is growing bigger. Let that happen slowly over a few minutes until the disc now fills the whole abdomino-pelvic space. Sit with the image for a while longer and notice how it affects your mind, body and Chi states. This is a powerful way to balance the Dan Tien and yin and yang throughout the body.

STAFF

Standing with your hands out in front of your chest and pelvis, imagine you are holding a wooden staff in your hands that runs along the length of the body in front of the spine. In the image, the staff does not touch the floor. Let your fingers curl around the image of the staff. As you settle into it and allow your body to become still, the staff will naturally start to align itself with your spine and central channels, so that you quite quickly experience a flow along the axis of your body. Play around with holding the staff in different places. Bringing the upper hand higher so that it holds the staff at head height can be very powerful. The hands are commonly placed in front of the Dan Tiens. Now imagine the staff touches the floor. What kind of Chi effect does that create? This is a wonderful meditation for gathering Chi to the core of the body and streamlining it. When the staff touches the floor it can act like an earthing rod, bringing your system into a more balanced and relaxed state.

SPHERE

Standing, imagine that at the centre of your chest there is a small sphere the size of a golf ball. Visualize that when you breathe in, some of your breath moves into the sphere, so that over a few breaths the sphere slowly begins to expand. Let this continue until the sphere fills the whole inside of the chest cavity. Pause here and just breathe in and out for a while, as if you were breathing in and out of the sphere. Now bring your hands up, so that your palms are looking at the centre of your chest, and your arms are rounded. Continue breathing and imagine the sphere expanding again, so that the sphere starts to expand out into the space formed by your hands and arms. Pause again when the sphere is the size of your arms and chest, just simply following your breath into the whole of this space. Let the sphere expand once more so that it feels as if it's pushing your hands and arms outwards. Let your hands and arms open out to accommodate this. The sphere keeps growing and expanding with your breath until your arms are pushed right out to the sides and the sphere sits on the floor and fills the whole space in front of you, up to head height and beyond. Pause again and be with the sense of space. Finally, bring your hands down to your middle Dan Tien, and step forward into the sphere so that you are completely within it. This should feel like a wonderful place of Chi. Let your mind and body rest and recharge in the sphere. You can repeat this exercise by starting with a sphere at the centre of your pelvis. It will produce a different space. This meditation is useful for getting to know your Dan Tiens more intimately and the fields they produce.

Chapter 15

CHI KUNG APPLICATIONS

ARTHRITIS

There's definitely no need for this condition when Chi Kung is available. Even when arthritis is in the family it can still be treated by Chi Kung practice. The solution is to keep your Chi moving. When it stops moving, your tissues shut down, in particular your connective tissue system. The "fascia" (the wrapping around muscles) becomes dense and loses its elastic, fluid quality. This condition migrates to the joint capsules and soon they follow suit, leading to more arthritic conditions.

Start with your spine. If your spine can move and be flexible and Chi can flow along the length of it, the rest of the body will follow. Do the swinging movements described in Chapter 1 (pages 19–23) under the section on the spine. Then spend time each day loosening your joints. (As described in Chapter 9.) Lastly, keep Chi moving along the length of the body to encourage flow from top to bottom. For persistent and painful joints, use your breath to move the Chi in the joints. So breathe into the joints every day. You can also make circular forms with your hands around any joint. Even if you are not close to it, you can use your intention.

LOW ENERGY

This is the disease of the modern era. Many people suffer from low energy and constantly feel fatigued. Even more people have bouts of exhaustion leading them to take time off work. Some people suffer from chronic fatigue, which can be so debilitating that you are unable to work and, in extreme cases, unable to look after yourself. Modern life is often stressful and pressurized and the body can become highly taxed. Long-term stress runs your body's natural resources down and in Chi Kung terms you lose your Jing, which is your constitutional energy handed down from your parents. This is not easy to replace, and some authorities in Chi Kung and Traditional Chinese Medicine believe it is not replaceable. However, anecdotal evidence suggests that people do make full recoveries from these states by serious practice of Chi Kung, change of diet and lifestyle.

An easy way to de-stress yourself is to slow your body down. Just doing Chi Kung forms allows this to happen; the slow movement forms and the internalization they evoke help your body's system move into a relaxed mode (a parasympathetic state). The more you do Chi Kung, the more you will switch your body off from its activated state. You will probably have been overriding your system for some time, so don't be surprised if you feel tired initially. Be careful of doing too much Chi Kung at first – try a couple of fifteen-minute sessions a day and that should suffice. Make sure you include joint opening exercises, as they will allow Chi to move more freely throughout your body.

One of the main indications of severe stress is that your body contracts, so the more you can open up and let the body expand, the better. It's important you include movements along the spine, as this will stimulate the Chi flow of the deeper, central channel and, once activated, this will regulate the whole energy system. Also make sure you include horizontal circular movements at the pelvis, waist, diaphragm and shoulders, as this will help relax the body and encourage Chi to free up from the body into the field around you, and vice versa. Always include Wu Chi stance in your practice. This will help ground the system, and settle the nervous system in particular; it will also reconnect the body to the earth, which in time will encourage a natural Chi flow into the body, re-energizing and revivifying everything.

IMPOTENCE

More and more men suffer from impotence. General health can be a major factor in this, so practising regular Chi Kung will strengthen your body and increase your Chi. The liver energy is commonly associated with sexual urges and this can, therefore, be worked with to increase the movement of Chi through the liver system.

The liver channel runs from the big toe up the inside of the leg and circles the sexual organs, then moves up the torso to the area of the liver. Try following this channel with your hands.

Bend forwards from your hips, with straight legs, and bring your hands in an arc out to the front of you so that the hands can sweep into the big toe. As you start to come upright, flex your knees to help your lower back, and move your hands up the inside of the legs. The hands don't touch the body, but remain a couple of inches away with the palms looking at the legs. When your hands reach the top of the legs, circle the hands around the sexual organs (both together in one direction, vary the direction on each repetition). Take the hands up past the liver along the length of the torso to the eyes and then take them forward in front of the eyes and back down to the feet in a big arc; then angle the hands forward as you bend once more and take the hands up the length of the channel. Repeat this each day, along with regular Chi Kung classes and practice, and it will increase your Chi flow.

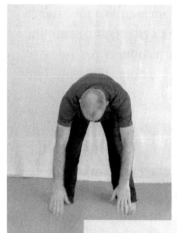

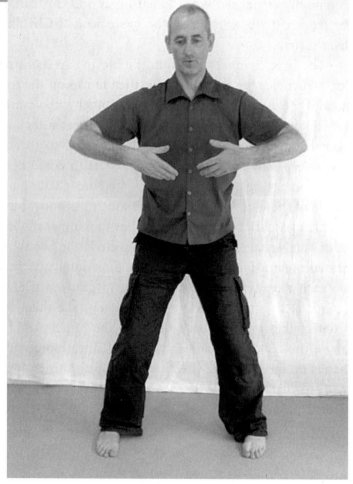

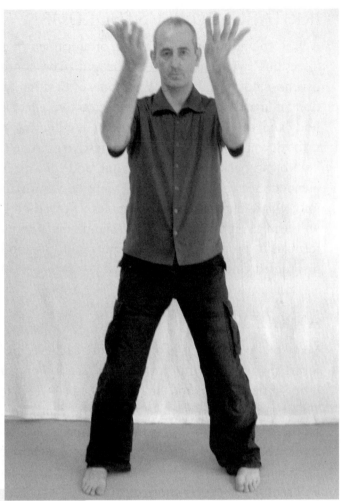

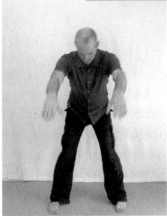

IRRITABLE BOWEL SYNDROME

A very common condition, this is often caused by stress or post-infectious hypersensitivity of the gut. The condition is often psycho-emotional, but the symptoms of bloating, pain, constipation or diarrhoea have a very destructive effect on the whole body and, especially if it is long-term, it will bring your Chi levels right down. There is a series of digestive exercise forms that can help bring balance back to the gut, and they are highly recommended. See the accompanying website www.naturalmovement. info, where there are many examples. If practised regularly, they will lead to an alleviation of the symptoms. The intention of the forms is to promote a fire in the guts and to smooth out chaotic, disordered Chi.

ANXIETY

Many of the symptoms of anxiety can be relieved by following the forms suggested in the "low energy" section on pages 163–164. It might be useful to add "shaking" (see pp.30–32) to those forms. This has a very powerful effect on the central nervous system. As the joints start to soften and decompress, especially along the spine, the nervous system literally has no choice but to relax. Even with long-term persistent anxiety patterns, regular practice will reduce the effects enormously.

HEADACHES

Headaches can be relieved by bringing Chi down from the head and facilitating a release of the Chi build-up. Start by loosening the joints in the shoulders and neck, then along the length of the spine by joint-opening exercises (see Chapter 9) and spinal swinging movements (see pp.19–23). Next make circular movements with your hands at the level of the cranial base, where the spine meets the head, for a few minutes. Do this by circling the hands out in front of your head. Make sure to rest your arms from time to time. Then take your hands to the level of the crown and make circular movements there too. Now bring your hands. palms upwards, up the sides of the body, right above the head, and slowly take the hands down the front of the body, palms leading. This will encourage Chi to move downwards towards the pelvis and to the feet. Keep this up for several minutes. At the end of it, keep your hands at your pelvis and simply point the centres of your palms to the centres of your feet and stay in this Wu Chi posture for a while.

ASTHMA

Many hyperallergenic conditions are becoming increasingly common, particularly asthma, which has increased dramatically over the last couple of decades, especially in children. It has been linked to many stress factors but, for children in particular, to stress from the mother. Chi Kung can help with this by relieving the symptoms. Allowing the chest to relax is the most important part of recovery. As the chest relaxes, the lungs reduce their contraction and then a normal state can return. Any movements that free up the chest will therefore encourage this. The two forms described below will help open the chest and free up the Chi there and along the lung channel. The lung channel runs from the thumb to the ribs down from the collarbones, along the inside of the arms.

Bring your fingertips to the centre of your breastbone, and let them hover just above the surface. (In Chi Kung there is rarely contact made with the body.) Start the movement at the bottom of the breastbone and, as you continue slowly, move upwards to the level of the collarbone. Draw out the hands across the chest to the sides and then forward into a circle, out in front of the chest. Then, as you bring the fingertips in towards the chest, breathe in, and keep breathing in till your hands have moved out

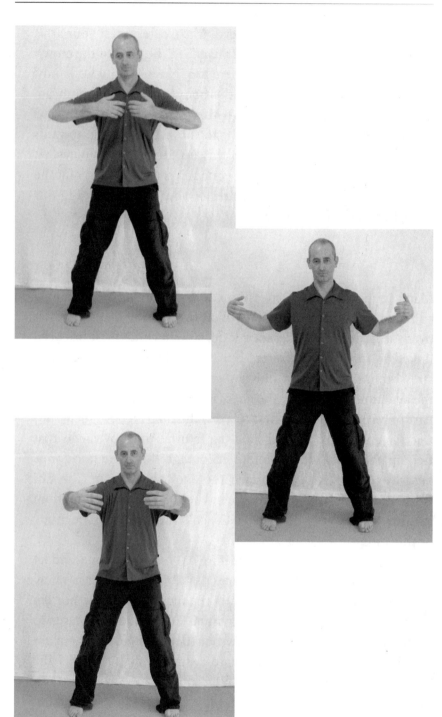

to the sides of the chest again. Sink as you breathe out and bring the hands forward in front of the chest.

In the second form, bring both palms close together out from the top of the chest, arms outstretched. Moving both arms together and keeping the whole movement at shoulder level, glide the palm of one hand along the length of the lung channel on the inside of the arm to the chest (without actually touching the arm). When you reach the chest, twist the outstretched arm and follow along the large intestine channel on the outside of the arm towards the first finger, as you bring your arms back to the front position. Now take the arms off to the other side and repeat.

The intention of the exercise is to stimulate the lung and large intestine channels, both of which are associated with the lungs and their Chi flow. As you repeat the movement form, try to make a smooth transition from left to right and let your centre of gravity shift with it. The hands do not touch the surface of the body, but glide a few inches above. For an instant the centres of the palms look at the first lung acupressure point near the collarbone. You will feel it, as it is a key energy gate in the body. Make sure your arms aren't locked straight. They need to be soft and pliable around each joint. As you continue, the channels will heat up and you should experience the lungs getting hot too. This is cleansing. At first you should make the movement for a few minutes, and then slowly, over a number of days, lengthen the time until you can make the movement for up to ten minutes.

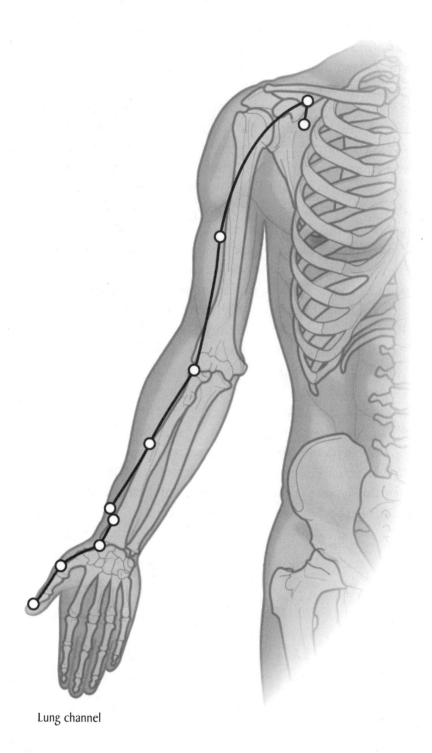

Lung channel

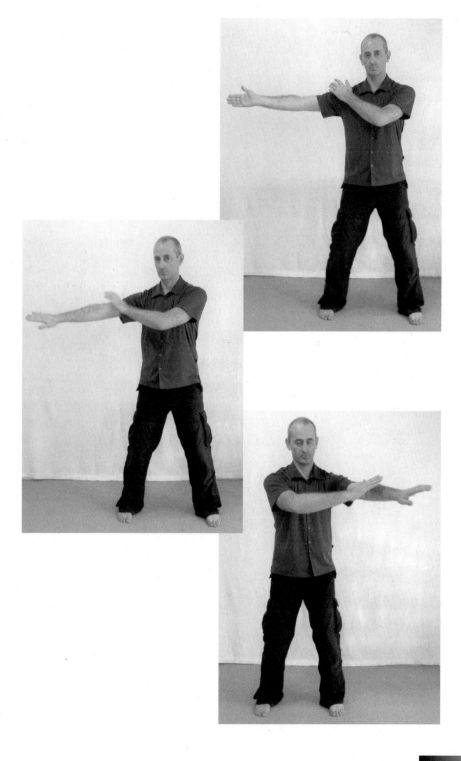

Meet Your Body
A Rolfer's Guide to Releasing Bodymindcore Trauma

Noah Karrasch

Paperback, ISBN 978 1 84819 016 0,
184 pages

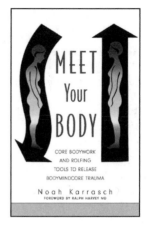

Many of us hold on to old fears, traumas and stresses and allow them to define and frame our lives. This book shows how to relieve these problems and help you look and feel better on a profound level. Based on the idea that the body is composed of twenty-one important hinges, *Meet Your Body* shows how we can 'oil' and free these hinges, stretching the body out so we can feel healthy and happy more of the time.

Noah's therapeutic work is influenced by his background in Rolfing, a hands-on manipulation of the body's connective tissue designed to enhance posture and freedom of movement. From this theory of structural integration, Karrasch has developed a focus on the inseparable connection between our minds and our bodies, our bodymindcore. Guiding the reader through the various hinges of the body, from the big toe to the hip to the head, the author shows how learning to isolate and stretch these hinges in new ways can lead to a happy bodymindcore, making a great difference to overall health and wellbeing. Each chapter addresses a particular hinge physically as well as sharing ideas about its emotional component, and includes photographs and drawings illustrating a variety of bodymindcore techniques.

This book offers people with both ordinary and extraordinary body challenges new ideas for how they can make changes in the way their bodies work for them. A practical guide to releasing bodymindcore trauma, *Meet Your Body* challenges us all to get in touch with and listen to our bodies to improve our health and overall happiness.

Breath in Action

The Art of Breath in Vocal and
Holistic Practice

Edited by Jane Boston and Rena Cook

Paperback, ISBN 978 1 84310 942 6,
256 pages

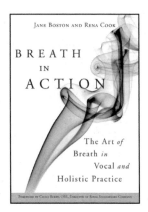

Breath in Action explores the significance of breath to human life, from the role it plays in communication to the more subtle ways it interacts with our voice and being. Offering the latest theories from a range of communicative and holistic fields, it shows that we can learn to breathe better so that, in turn, we may communicate better, act better, sing better, and feel better.

A group of leading practitioners and theorists from the arts, the healing arts, and the speech and medical sciences explore ways in which the conscious use and management of breath can enhance health, creativity, and performance. Their insights combine personal narratives and historical scholarship with practice-based evidence and easy-to-follow breathing exercises. Each section of the book looks in detail at a different aspect of breath: breath in the body, breath and the mind, breath and holistic practice, and breath and performance. Together they show that deep, mindful breathing can spread calmness, power and vitality throughout the mind, body and soul, and provide a means of transforming one's voice and one's self.

Breath in Action is a comprehensive guide to the potency, impact and authority of breath, as well as to its many applications in the communicative and holistic fields. It is required reading for voice and speech trainers, performers, professional speakers, holistic practitioners, and anyone else wishing to master the art of breath.